When the City Stopped

When the City Stopped

Stories from New York's Essential Workers

Robert W. Snyder

Three Hills
an imprint of Cornell University Press
Ithaca and London

First published 2025 by Cornell University Press

Printed in the United States of America

Library of Congress Cataloging-in-Publication Data

Names: Snyder, Robert W., 1955– author.

Title: When the city stopped : stories from New York's essential workers / Robert W. Snyder.

Description: Ithaca : Cornell University Press, 2025. | Includes bibliographical references and index.

Identifiers: LCCN 2024028893 (print) | LCCN 2024028894 (ebook) | ISBN 9781501780387 (paperback) | ISBN 9781501780400 (epub) | ISBN 9781501780394 (pdf)

Subjects: LCSH: COVID-19 Pandemic, 2020—New York (State)–New York. | COVID-19 Pandemic, 2020—Social aspects–New York (State)–New York. | LCGFT: Personal narratives.

Classification: LCC RA644.C67 S6224 2025 (print) | LCC RA644.C67 (ebook) | DDC 616.2/41440097471–dc23/eng/20240904

LC record available at https://lccn.loc.gov/2024028893

LC ebook record available at https://lccn.loc.gov/2024028894

*In memory of all who were lost and
In honor of the frontline workers who
faced danger so that the rest of us
might live.*

Contents

Editor's Note

The oral history interviews in this book were conducted by the Bronx COVID-19 Oral History Project at Fordham University; the NYC COVID-19 Oral History, Narrative, and Memory Project at Columbia University; the Queens Memory Project; the Staten Island Coronavirus Chronicle at the College of Staten Island; and by Martha Guerrero Badillo and myself. I edited the interviews for length and clarity, and then reviewed them with their narrators to ensure that my editing had not distorted their meanings.

—Robert W. Snyder

When the City Stopped

Introduction

In the spring of 2020, during the darkest days of the COVID-19 pandemic, New York City was silent. Streets were empty. At its worst, close to eight hundred people were dying every day.[1] Riding a subway or walking past a stranger, everyday tests of urban sociability, seemed to become matters of life and death. Would someone's cough infect you with COVID-19, setting off a catastrophic cascade of events that would lead you to die alone in a hospital bed? There was no way to know. All who could worked online or huddled at home. Direct human connections, the oxygen of city life, carried the threat of mortal danger.

This book, based on oral histories, first-person narratives, and poetry from New Yorkers who lived through the pandemic, tells the stories of how New Yorkers not only suffered, but—in acts of solidarity great and small—coped and worked to help the city recover. Small gestures accumulated, direct ties forged larger bonds, and in the work of people as varied as clergy, retail workers, nurses, doctors, EMTs, and restaurant owners, I glimpsed a little-recognized truth of the pandemic: in the days when New York felt abandoned and besieged, it was saved from the bottom up. How this solidarity was built, along with its strengths and limitations, must be remembered and understood if we are to fully fathom the history of the pandemic and grasp what needs to be done better in the next public health emergency.

Nothing in the city's recent history prepared anyone for the full onslaught of COVID-19. The cholera epidemics of the nineteenth century and the global flu epidemic of 1918 had been forgotten by the general public. The AIDS epidemic of the 1980s, while devastating for the gay community, did not immediately threaten the entire population the way COVID-19 would. The terrorist attacks of September 11, 2001, were deadly, but with the exception of first responders who died lingering deaths from breathing toxic smoke, ash and debris, the carnage was limited to one terrible day. International cooperation contained SARS (Severe Acute Respiratory Syndrome) in 2003 and left people confident in public health authorities.[2]

New York City had a robust system of public and private hospitals and a Department of Health with a nationally recognized reputation. It also had a long history of effective public health campaigns: the nineteenth-century sanitary reformers whose works created a cleaner and healthier city; the public health clinics of the Progressive and New Deal eras; the mass vaccination campaigns against smallpox and polio after World War II; and the successful efforts to reduce smoking during the Bloomberg mayoralty. The city seemed well positioned to face the challenge of COVID-19.[3]

The pandemic, however, would reveal a more troubling reality. Since the fiscal crisis of 1975, New York had slashed the robust commitment to public welfare on a social democratic scale that had once defined the city. Hospitals were closed in Harlem, the South Bronx, and Brooklyn. Many hospitals reduced their number of beds for a variety of reasons, including a shift from inpatient to outpatient care made possible by improvements in drugs and surgical techniques and the growth of hospice care at home. Hospitals received varying reimbursements from Medicare, Medicaid, and private insurers—leaving hospitals serving the poor with fewer resources than those with a mix of patients. This set the stage for extreme challenges when the pandemic hit. The city maintained public hospitals, but these had weaker funding than elite private hospitals. In areas inhabited by people of color, working-class people, and immigrants—where overcrowded housing made for the rapid transmission of communicable diseases—financially strained hospitals lacked the capacity to treat a large influx of patients. In a city once famous for its ability to manufacture clothing, the departure of garment manufacturing left hospitals dependent on global supply chains for basic equipment like masks and protective clothing. And then came the COVID-19 pandemic.[4]

By April 2020 a month of lockdowns and wailing sirens made it clear that the city's institutions were ill-equipped to handle the emergency. Hospitals set up refrigerated trucks to hold the bodies of the dead while overwhelmed funeral homes struggled to cope.

At an online meeting of historians, archivists, folklorists, and documentarians, Josh Brown of the American Social History Project suggested that COVID-19 would be a historic event on the scale of the Great Depression in the 1930s. With that thought in mind, many of us took steps to document the unfolding disaster for future generations. We were determined to avoid the unfathomable precedent of the last great pandemic to sweep New York city, the flu of 1918, which took some thirty thousand lives but was not marked by a single memorial and left no long-term impact on public consciousness. The AIDS epidemic and terrorist attacks of 9/11 had their memorials, but as precedents neither aligned perfectly with COVID-19.[5]

Oral historians at Columbia University, the College of Staten Island, Fordham University, and the Queens Memory Project organized interviews that could be conducted online and by telephone to eliminate the danger of getting infected with COVID-19 at an in-person interview. Archivists at Brooklyn College, the New York Historical Society, the Schomburg Center, and the Museum of the City of New York began to collect first-person narratives, photographs, paintings, digital resources, and objects from everyday life under COVID-19. The folklorists at City Lore launched a group poem and collected oral histories, poems, young people's responses to the pandemic, signs, song parodies, and memorials to the dead. Historians Ellen Noonan at New York University and Peter Aigner at the Gotham Center for New York City History at CUNY set up websites to exchange ideas about working through the crisis and to document the many COVID-19-related projects that appeared in New York City alone. All these efforts produced a trove of sources that will be mined for years to come to produce many books, articles, films, and exhibits on COVID-19 in New York City.[6]

It was too soon to attempt a history of the disaster, but the right time to compile people's first impressions for future generations. As Manhattan Borough Historian, I wanted to produce a book that would ensure that the experiences of New Yorkers during the pandemic were not forgotten. With help from Gracia Brown and Brendan Reynolds, I started to read transcripts of the interviews that were being conducted around the city with the goal of publishing a selection from them in a book.

After many months of reading, I dug into the more difficult job of selecting what to publish. My goal was not to produce an encyclopedia of experiences that was statistically representative of all New Yorkers, but a record of illuminating lives and memories. Again and again, I was drawn to interviews and poems that got at the depth and complexity of people living and working in hard times: a man who lived through the AIDS epidemic who drew on the lessons of that plague to work at a hospital through COVID-19; an immigrant paramedic who learned to take calculated risks as a mountaineer and likes to work in low-income neighborhoods that need his services; a restaurant owner who delivered food to locked-down customers and provided them with not just meals but human contact. Then I conducted interviews of my own to round out the range of experiences presented, especially among transit workers and uniformed first responders.

The stories of COVID-19 survivors and the stories of people who lost loved ones to COVID-19 were poignant. Survivors who contracted COVID-19 sometimes went to a hospital and lingered for days in a shadowland between life and death. Those who lost friends or family to COVID-19 were haunted by the thought that their loved one died alone, their last earthly sensations carried to them through a cell phone, held up next to their death bed by an obliging nurse. People coped with loneliness and loss. They learned to persevere and share their burdens in the hopes of someday emerging from the pandemic whole and healed as both individuals and as a city.

But the goal of surviving, in both a medical and a civic sense, was advanced most by the people who—paid or unpaid—went out and worked. Their stories are at the heart of this book. Knowingly exposing themselves to the dangers of the pandemic they drove buses, ran subways, answered 911 calls, tended to the sick, erected memorials to the dead, and made and delivered meals. Individually and collectively, they affirmed the bonds between New Yorkers and kept the city functioning.

New Yorkers were "alone together," in a morale-boosting phrase of the day. Yet they were separated by both the protective measures of social distancing and the fundamental realities of life and work in New York City: it was immigrants, people with low incomes, and people of color who were more likely to do jobs that required face-to-face contact in the city's service, retail, and transit sectors and more likely to go home to crowded housing where the virus spread easily.[7]

Relatively well-off New Yorkers could stay safe within the confines of their private apartments and order takeout food or, if they were sufficiently affluent, retreat to their country houses. It was far more dangerous for a delivery worker to spend endless hours on a bicycle delivering takeout food to multiple customers, and then go home to an apartment with three generations of family members to wrestle with the fact that they might be carrying the virus that would kill their grandmother.

COVID-19 made connecting with other people awkward at best and dangerous at worst. Still, New Yorkers found ways to reach out to one another to cope, to mourn, and to perform the unheralded jobs that are essential to keeping the city running.

In an age when so much of reality is understood as "virtual," they faced actual hardships in the streets, on subways, in stores, and in hospitals. Their work affirmed a point made by the literary critic Paul Fussell: there are only two classes of people—those who might get hurt or killed on the job and those who won't.[8] The pandemic dramatically expanded the number of jobs that carried a mortal risk, then doubled the inequality by disproportionately claiming the lives of Black and Brown New Yorkers.

Faced with such dangers—more than forty-five thousand New Yorkers and more than a million Americans died of COVID-19 from 2020 to 2023—people who worked under the threat of COVID-19 were sustained by many different beliefs and values. Medical workers, firefighters, and police officers were strengthened by professional ideals of courage and service. Others who

worked for the common good were fortified by class consciousness, religion, pride in work, and a desire to sustain their neighbors. Still others worked because they had no alternative: they had
rent to pay or families to support.[9]

Just as COVID-19 touched all aspects of people's lives, from
ideas about politics to how we approached grocery shopping, New
Yorkers drew on different corners of their lives and selves to meet
COVID-19's challenges. In the interviews, poems, and narratives
that I studied, conducted, and selected, one of the most prominent
themes was solidarity: where it comes from, what sustains it, and
what it can accomplish. There is a venerable tradition of writing
about solidarity in times of crisis. Rebecca Solnit has argued that
the spontaneous generosity that occurs during disasters reveals
our better selves, makes us our brothers' and sisters' keepers, and
can create what her book title calls *A Paradise Built in Hell*.[10] There
was much of this in COVID-19, from the people who sewed protective masks when they were in desperately short supply to the
young people who helped their elders wrangle vaccine appointments from badly designed vaccination registration websites.

Solidarity, however, came up against limits. There were heroic
examples of mutual aid in New York City during the pandemic,
but neighborhood action programs acting alone could not produce the vaccines needed to stem the spread of the virus. Volunteers have an important role to play in facing long-term crises, but
we also need professionals who can engage them full time. If we
are to do better in future public health emergencies, we need to
reconcile the tensions between professionalism and voluntarism
to produce the best possible mixture of both.

And the story of the pandemic in New York City was not entirely
a story of solidarity. National political divisions leached into local
debates over masking, vaccines, and the best ways to bring people

back together after the deadly surge of spring 2020. The origins of the virus in China led to anti-Asian violence, attacks on Jews rose during the pandemic, and the Black Lives Matter demonstrations responding to the murder of George Floyd in May 2020 illuminated protestors and police bitterly at odds with each other. Once vaccines were introduced and COVID-19 became less lethal, there was less foxhole solidarity. Demonstrations against vaccine mandates for municipal workers occurred in lower Manhattan, and restaurant workers were troubled by customers who showed no enthusiasm for mask mandates.

By May 11, 2023, when federal authorities declared the COVID-19 public health emergency ended, New Yorkers—like their ancestors after the flu of 1918—were entering a state of collective amnesia, forgetting things that had happened to them only a few years before. But memory can help us prepare for the future, especially when it helps us understand the best of human responses to a crisis. "People need to hear," Vaclav Havel once wrote, "that it

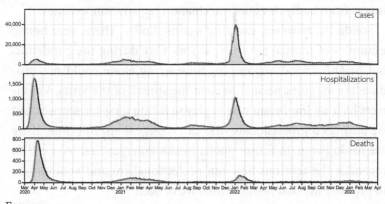

FIGURE 1
COVID-19 in New York City: Total cases, hospitalizations, and deaths, March 2020 to April 2023. Chart: BetaNYC. Data: New York City Department of Health and Mental Hygiene.

makes sense to behave decently or to help others, to place common interests above their own, to respect the elementary rules of human coexistence."[11]

Against forgetting, ignorance, and disinformation, this book sets down individual memories, confirmed facts, and a wide range of experiences. Here are the words of forty-five New Yorkers who struggled through the COVID-19 pandemic. Their contributions are organized both thematically and chronologically, from the eve of the pandemic emergency in early 2020 to its official end three years later.

In reflecting on their passage through the pandemic, these contributors left for future generations a record of courage, heartache, strength, wisdom, and compassion. If you find some surprises or inspiration in their words, this book will have done its job.

Their stories begin on the eve of the pandemic, in the early months 2020. Even as terrifying reports of the virus causing mass deaths in Italy reached New York City, many New Yorkers gathered in crowds as if somehow their city would escape the worst.

1

Early Days, Winter 2020

On March 2, 2020, the day after New York State recorded its first confirmed case of COVID-19, Governor Andrew Cuomo appeared in Manhattan with Mayor Bill de Blasio and medical and civic leaders to reassure people that even as the coronavirus was devastating China and Italy, their state and city were not in danger. "We have the best health care system in the world here," he said. "And excuse our arrogance as New Yorkers, I speak for the Mayor also on this one, we think we have the best health care system on the planet right here in New York. So, when you're saying what happened in other countries versus what happened here, we don't think it's going to be as bad as it was in other countries."[1]

The following years proved his optimism wrong. More than forty-five thousand New Yorkers would die, despite the city's excellent hospitals and its health department. The pandemic would wreck the city's economy, disrupt its schools for years, and tear at its social fabric.[2]

As historians of public health, medicine, and disasters have made clear, epidemics are much more than germs and viruses set in motion. Epidemics gain force and significance in their context, in communities, cities, states, and nations. They exploit and expose inequalities that leave some people more vulnerable than others. The coronavirus may have originated in China, but the way that it wracked New York City was made in America and lived out in New York. From the federal government to local officials, the pandemic was defined by failures of leadership. And in the streets, transit system, and homes of New York City, the coronavirus spread and infected on a devastating scale.[3]

COVID-19 struck the United States when it was already in the depths of what the historian Daniel T. Rodgers has called the "age of fracture," a period when the ideas about politics, identities, societies, and institutions that had once held the United States together fragmented, to be replaced by a cacophony of claims connected only by a deep faith in the market. At the top of the federal government, President Donald Trump—presiding over a country deeply polarized by regional and political identities—announced that the virus would someday vanish, speculated in public on medically preposterous cures, put money into the development of vaccines, and attacked elected officials, journalists, and public health authorities who questioned his actions. To be sure, there were strengths within federal agencies and individuals who met the pandemic with courage and high standards of professionalism, but these could not overcome a general lack of preparedness and operational capabilities in the federal government. But the confusion wrought by the Trump White House reverberated nationally, undermining the credibility of federal officials, and weakening the effectiveness of government responses to a national problem.[4]

The situation was little better at lower levels of government. In matters of public health, the federalist structure of government in the United States devolves considerable autonomy to fifty states and more than three thousand counties. Faced with a pandemic that could travel with the speed of a continental jet flight, this devolution made it difficult to coordinate any national strategy against COVID-19—even if there had been one. In theory, decentralization left open the possibility of crafting local responses to specific circumstances, but in practice it led to an ever-changing patchwork of city, county, and state policies on matters such as masking, business closures, and stay-at-home orders that undermined public confidence in government and may have increased the spread of the virus. Moreover, poorly funded state and local public health departments were ill-equipped to overcome the long-standing inequalities that made Black and Latino people more vulnerable to infection and less likely to receive adequate care.[5]

COVID-19 also struck in what has been described as the "neoliberal" era, a period from the 1970s onward when free market capitalism was acclaimed as the best way to organize societies, ensure human freedom, and deliver prosperity. In contrast to the earlier New Deal order, which stressed the power of government and regulation to shape the economy in ways that delivered a broad prosperity, neoliberalism applauded market systems and market-based outcomes. The global recession of 2008–9 shook faith in neoliberalism, but as late as 2020 it remained a strong force in the United States and in both the Democratic and Republican parties.[6]

Neoliberalism reshaped New York, but the city brought significant strengths to confront coronavirus—a labor movement that was stronger than in most American cities, public and private hospitals, a proud tradition of municipal public health work embodied in its Department of Health and Mental Hygiene, an activist disposition, and a sense of its own grit that was confirmed in New York's recovery from the terrorist attacks of September 11, 2001. Since the days of the Progressive Era and the New Deal, there was also an enduring belief—however bruised by periodic budget cuts and narrowing definitions of the public good—that public health was the birthright of all New Yorkers.[7]

The populous and powerful city of New York might have appeared to be well positioned to meet the challenges of COVID-19, but as the course of the pandemic would show, it was deeply vulnerable. As a global city with direct transportation links to the rest of the world, New York received COVID-19 via international airline flights—primarily from Europe.

New York in 2020 was also, however, a city with significant inequalities. Middle-class and affluent New Yorkers with good health insurance could rely on some of the best hospitals in the world, almost all of them run by health corporations. Poor and low-income New Yorkers, who often lacked health insurance, were prone to relying on municipally owned hospitals that were not as well funded as their corporate counterparts.[8]

Black, Brown, and lower-income New Yorkers lived and worked in circumstances that made them more vulnerable to disease and chronic health problems. At work, they were more likely to labor in settings that put them in direct contact with the public—as transit workers, cashiers, retail store staff, service workers, or hospital staff.[9]

And their city was an increasingly expensive place to live in, setting off a chain of consequences that made them more vulnerable to the virus. Population growth outpaced the construction of affordable housing, and poor, working-class, and middle-class New Yorkers found it ever harder to cover housing costs. In Brooklyn and Queens, the two boroughs with the largest immigrant populations, multiple generations often lived together in crowded housing.

Perhaps most important, the disease spread asymptomatically and faster than anyone imagined. In early March, when Governor Cuomo announced that New Yorkers would do better than other places afflicted with the virus, the absence of adequate testing muddied full knowledge of the extent of COVID-19's presence in the New York metropolitan area. Indeed, subsequent research shows that COVID-19 was in New York City as early as January and was circulating rapidly by early March.[10]

In the days and weeks after Cuomo's announcement, COVID-19 spread through the city. The governor and mayor—in one more episode of their dangerously cantankerous fight for dominance— disagreed over what to do. On March 5, the mayor rode the subway to reassure New Yorkers that it was safe. Privately health department officials were alarmed. When the mayor on March 17 said New Yorkers should be ready to "shelter in place" to protect themselves from the virus, Governor Cuomo said the mayor was overstepping his authority.[11]

On March 20, with Broadway closed, schools closed, and refrigerator trucks set up outside hospitals to handle an anticipated overflow of dead bodies, the governor announced his "New York on Pause" plan, which would take effect March 22. Under it, all nonessential workers were required to stay at home, nonessential businesses were required to close, and New Yorkers over seventy were required to stay at home. New York was now a city under lockdown at the epicenter of a global pandemic.[12]

Fear, Hygiene, and Teaching

Damien LaRock

Damien LaRock lives in Douglaston, Queens, and works as a special education teacher at P.S. 148 in East Elmhurst, Queens. When he first heard about COVID-19 in January 2020, he was in a taxi; the driver had the radio tuned to 1010 WINS, and a story came on about a new virus spreading in China.[13]

LATE JANUARY OR early to mid-February I took a field trip with my class to the Queens Botanical Garden. We were riding the school bus and one of my students, Reinaldo, asked me what the coronavirus was. So we started to talk about it, and he started to express some fear that he heard that this virus was going to come here. And I remember trying to think really carefully about how to respond to him because, you know, he's a nine-year-old child, and I certainly didn't want to make him feel worried about it, but I also didn't want to give him a false sense of comfort. So I just tried to explain what I knew about the virus.

But after that it definitely became more and more present in our daily consciousness every single day. The kids were talking about it more in school. I remember my coteacher and I, and several friends who were teachers, started having more and more conversations about what was going to happen if the virus were to come to New York City.

I had a conversation with my coteacher about needing to do some lessons with our kids about washing their hands and covering their coughs. And these are third graders. So we knew that this was going to be a struggle. We had lots of conversations about finding this tricky balance between teaching hygiene, making sure that we were talking about the virus, but also not instilling too much fear in our kids.

The Angel of Death over Italy

Fabio Girelli-Carasi

In the New York metropolitan area, an ethnically diverse region in a global media system, it was possible to watch COVID-19 wreak devastation overseas and anticipate its eventual impact on New York. One who watched the progress of COVID-19 in Italy closely was Fabio Girelli-Carasi, a professor of Modern Languages and Literatures at Brooklyn College.[14]

MY IMMEDIATE FAMILY, sister and mother, live in the city of Albino, in the province of Bergamo, the hardest hit area in Italy. The rest of my family lives in Cremona, the second hardest hit area in Italy.

My sister contracted the virus at the very beginning of the pandemic, sometime in February 2020, before the lockdown began. She locked herself up in her room for six weeks and eventually recovered. Six months later she still suffers from fatigue and on-and-off muscle pain. Two older relatives of mine died from the virus. One was in a hospital for minor surgery he had postponed for a few months. When he finally decided to get it done, it was right at the beginning of the storm. He was infected and died in a matter of days. The second one was in assisted living. The angel of death glided over the facility and took more than two dozen residents with it.

The most painful was the death of a high school friend, a family doctor in Como. He started seeing patients with strange symptoms. With no guidance and no information from the Ministry of Health, he kept doing his job. When he came down with the infection, the viral load was so high he only lasted a few days.

My mother escaped the infection. She lives in the same building as my sister, but they didn't see each other for months. She lived alone like a recluse. Friends or relatives would drop off food by her door, she would put out the garbage and that was it. In the meantime, she kept hearing stories of people she had known for a lifetime who were passing away: "They are dropping like flies" she told me one day. She mentioned a famous poem by Italian poet Giuseppe Ungaretti, which he wrote while he was fighting in the trenches of World War I: "We are like leaves on a branch in autumn."

I spent hours every day, sometimes several times a day for weeks, trying to console and give her courage. At a certain point I thought she was about to give up. She wasn't eating anymore, she was getting weaker and weaker, half asleep the whole day, awake in terror and sorrow at night.

As to my life, it is similar to that of most of you. I live outside New York City, my wife, two daughters and I managed with some adjustments in our routines. I avoided social networks like the plague (sorry for the metaphor,) stayed away from the news and commentaries, focused on my teaching as much as possible, even took care of the backyard.

Over the months, it became discouraging to the point of banging my head on my desk as I was watching Europe slowly getting control over the pandemic, while in the United States we were and still are stumbling like blind morons, clueless and bamboozled by borderline criminal propaganda.

Of course, not everybody fits this profile, but frankly, it is horrifying and terrifying to know that every other person I see in the streets lives in a state of willful derangement, posing a danger to themselves (even if I could care less about them) but most of all to the rest of us.

Looming Threats to Transit Workers

Re'gan Weal

Re'gan Weal grew up on the Lower East Side of Manhattan in an African American family of transit workers. Her grandfather was a dispatcher, and in 2006 she followed in her mother's footsteps to become a bus operator. She is a member of Local 100 of the Transport Workers Union. When COVID-19 hit, she was on the M20 route from Lincoln Center at 63rd Street and Broadway to South Ferry.[15]

IT'S NOT THE easiest job. I have a love–hate relationship with it, let's just put it that way. I love driving. But it has its moments, the people make it hard at times. The traffic, depending on what route you're on, can be a little rough—especially during rush hour. But other than that, it's a pretty great job.

Around December 2019 you heard little things here and there. You didn't really hear more about it until January. And then in February things started getting a little weird in the city. Then when March came around, everything just shut down.

The MTA wasn't on board with people wearing masks. They said it wasn't part of the uniform. So they weren't allowing us to wear a mask at the time.

It was when it was reported on the news that people were dying that they said okay. But they didn't have a supply of masks for us. We had to supply ourselves. Eventually, they provided us with masks and then made it mandatory. But it wasn't right away.

Our union, TWU Local 100, fought for us to have PPE, to have some sort of protection, even though transit was against it. They were able to win the battle and get us what we needed to work in a safe environment.

At some point transit decided to put COVID-19 cleaners on the bus. And they would have people come clean the buses at our layovers or when we're switching operators. They did put some protection in place after they realized it was really bad, but you kind of wonder, was it too late?

We usually wipe our buses down anyway because you just never know. But at that time we were very diligent about it. We would all try to have Lysol or Lysol wipes, or Bleach Wipes, to wipe down the bus.

We wiped everything that someone could possibly touch because we didn't know at that time how you could contract COVID-19.

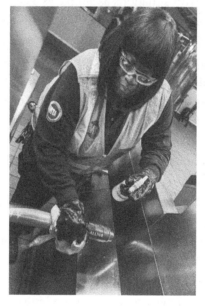

FIGURE 2
Early in the pandemic, the Metropolitan Transit Authority set workers to scrubbing subway stations. It turned out that airborne transmissions were much more dangerous than infected surfaces. Photograph by Patrick Cashin, MTA.

The Start of a Pandemic

Ali Mazinov

Ali Mazinov, a health sciences major at Brooklyn College, immigrated to the United States from Russia with his family at the age of four and has since then lived in Brooklyn, first in Sunset Park and later in Midwood.[16]

I WORKED AS a New York City paramedic for several years before the COVID-19 pandemic hit the world. As paramedics, we were trained to deal with situations as simple as a cut on the arm or as complex as directing a team to care for a cardiac arrest patient.

When COVID-19 hit New York City, I was unaware of how bad it was going to get. At first, we thought it was a virus that was weaker than influenza, which is something we deal with on a regular basis. At this time, we would get one call a day that was related to COVID-19. I thought that everyone was exaggerating.

Over time, COVID-19 patients became more frequent, and in the matter of a month it was the only type of call we would get. It was as if every other medical problem that people had went away. But this was because everyone that wasn't infected with COVID-19 was too afraid to go to the hospital.

When things started to take a turn for the worse, people were starting to go into life-threatening conditions on each call. My partner and I would need to resort to extreme measures like putting a tube down a person's windpipe and into their lungs to help them breathe. Sometimes this wouldn't be enough, and the patient would go into cardiac arrest from the lack of oxygen in the body.

It was a very difficult time for me because I felt powerless to stop people from dying from this terrible disease. It got so bad that the hospitals did not have the capacity to accept any more patients that came in. People were put in hallways, next to nursing stations, and hospitals had to dedicate entire floors to COVID-19 patients.

Then another problem started to rear its head. My co-workers and friends started to get sick. Those of us with families had to make a choice, either quit their job to protect their families or live apart from them until this was all over.

We did not have enough EMT's and paramedics to staff the ambulances we had running on any given day. Those of us who were not sick picked up anywhere from sixty to ninety hours a week.

This struggle continues now as well. All over the world, there are not enough emergency services personnel to cope with the call volume that we are given each day.

A Weird State

Keerthan Thiyagarajah

Keerthan Thiyagarajah was born and raised in Queens in a Sri Lankan family. He was living in Jackson Heights, studying culinary management at LaGuardia Community College, and commuting to Manhattan to work as a cook when the pandemic began.[17]

IT WAS A weird state in New York and everywhere in general. Nobody knew what to do. There was toilet paper flying off the shelves, water bottles, people price gouging. It was impossible to get anything you needed. People were selling hand sanitizer on Amazon for like six hundred dollars a bottle. When people were at their weakest, people thought they could just make a profit off people's weaknesses and the general public's health.

Luckily for me, my parents, for some reason, loved to store tons and tons of toilet paper in our pantry. So that was nothing to be worried about. But when it comes to gloves, KN95 masks, and stuff like that, that's where I think a lot of people lacked because it's something we don't prepare for.

Some of the lasting memories I had during those months, early February going into March: I remember governments telling us, "Hey, stay indoors, wear a mask, do everything you can to just stay home. We're going to close down schools, we're going to do this and we're going to try to remediate."

Davidson Garrett

Davidson Garrett, a poet, writer, and actor who lives in the NoMad section of Manhattan on East 28th Street, drove a taxi in New York City from 1978 to 2018.[18]

early morning fog
covers the town like a shroud
death floats in the air

Worrying for the City

Jessica B. Martinez

Jessica B. Martinez, a global health expert with a background in virology and infectious diseases, lives in the Hamilton Heights section of Manhattan with her husband. She first heard rumblings about COVID-19 in December 2019, and as February 2020 gave way to March, the situation around her grew more dire.[19]

I WAS JUST worried for the city.

The last part of March and the early part of April were just awful. Just—wow. [*crying*] Sorry. Constant sirens. You know, just that constant—it's either deathly quiet or it is a hundred percent sirens.

I lost a couple of former colleagues from my old company, and a couple of neighbors who were older and weren't really able to fight the virus.

Cuomo did a great job, I think, in terms of getting everybody on the same page very quickly, and the "Keep calm and carry on" discussion. Maybe he could have done a few things differently with the nursing homes and things like that. But in the grand scheme of things, it was terrible and it was awful.

The first week of April was when we peaked here and my birthday's April 8 so I just remember thinking, awesome, this is going to be a great way to think about your birthday for the rest of your life.

Her professional view

In a lot of ways, I feel like I've been kind of anticipating a pandemic for most of my life. I don't know how many twelve-year-olds know what an epidemiologist is, but I did, and I wanted to be one.

From a virologist's perspective, and this is going to sound so sick, it is one of the most fascinating viruses I think I've ever seen and heard of. It's just so weird, it does such weird things. It doesn't behave the way that we expect most viruses to work, and we still don't even know what it does.

So I also feel like I probably have a front-row seat to all the horror that the virus can cause—you know, all the different ways it can cause your body to go haywire—and that also made it really difficult to just think about all these people. And I've got to say, seeing Hart Island and all those morgue trucks—I never thought I'd see mass graves.

The Sirens

Led Black

Led Black, a New York–born writer, grew up in the Washington Heights section of Manhattan with close ties to the Dominican Republic. When COVID-19 struck New York City, his blog at www. uptowncollective.com turned to local and national dimensions of the pandemic. On April 2, he addressed the noise that defined the city's darkest days: the sound of sirens.[20]

I FALL ASLEEP to sirens. I wake up to sirens. The sirens are incessant. The sirens, at least in New York City, are the soundtrack to this pandemic. The sirens are constant and what you start to realize after spending every waking moment dealing with the nerve-racking sirens is that what you are hearing is not a single siren at a time but multiple, different sirens simultaneously. The lament of the ambulance fighting with the cop car and the fire truck for dominance and winning. The sirens are the city wailing out in despair. The night is upon us like never before, but this too shall pass.

Well, you have to keep telling yourself that at least. This is really, really scary. This thing is heavy like "is this the end times?" heavy. It is hard to not succumb to despair, gloom and doom when you realize that the absolutely feckless and moronic Trump, who is in way over his head in this situation, is the current occupant of the Oval Office and the most powerful man on the planet. You can't tweet diss the pandemic away. Trump bet the farm that this would be a mild illness that would be gone by April, and we are now paying the price for his madness and colossal ineptitude. In short order, Donald Trump has turned the United States into a s-hole country.

This is America. We should not be where we are right now. For such a great country to be brought down so low because of a lack of foresight, vision, and planning is inexcusable. This is what happens when a failed, racist in decline, reality TV personality becomes the president. Leadership matters. Intelligence matters. Judgment matters. Empathy matters. Donald Trump fails on all counts.

The world has changed overnight, and the very notion of certainty has become a cruel joke. Our FB feeds speak of folks losing loved ones quickly and unexpectedly. My wife is keeping a running list of friends and family that have contracted the virus that is up to twenty-three and growing fast. One death in that twenty-three. Our prayers, condolences, and love go out to all who are feeling the impact of the novel coronavirus.

Miss Rona [COVID], like my eldest daughter likes to call her, is exposing the holes in a society that has for far too long put profit before people. New York City is hurting and about to be at a breaking point.

But we will not break. We shall overcome but things can never be the same again. The status quo is not going to cut it anymore. A better world is possible. Let's work together to build it.

Pa'Lante Siempre Pa'Lante!

Lamb's Blood

Steve Zeitlin

The folklorist Steve Zeitlin recalls that when he wrote "Lamb's Blood" in May 2020, "fear was a way of life." He was in his early seventies, immunocompromised, and—though rarely given to thoughts of religion—faced with a pandemic of biblical proportions. "The last verse has the quality of a prayer," he wrote later. "Prayers, as a rabbi once put it, open us up to the healing powers that God has already placed in the universe. Prayers aplenty can ground us as we confront a situation in which we have limited control."[21]

The Jews have seen it all –
waters of the Nile turned blood red
frogs
lice
flies
pestilence
boils
hail
locusts
darkness
and the killing of the firstborn child.

But now
the world is quarantined
as if an X in lamb's blood
were drawn upon all our doors.

May this plague spare us all –
the good people of the planet –
Christian, Hindu, Muslim, Jew.

May the Angel of Death pass over our houses
May the Red Sea part.
May cities and towns reopen.
May we all pass through.

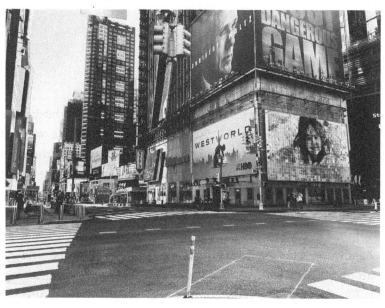

FIGURE 3
May 2020: When Governor Andrew Cuomo put New York on pause in
March 2020, busy neighborhoods like Times Square became ghost towns until
late May. Photograph by Arlene Schulman.

2

Working for the Public's Health, Spring 2020

When Governor Cuomo ordered all nonessential businesses to close March 22, 2020, he divided the city's workers into two categories: those who would face the danger of the virus directly and those who could work from home in relative safety. Most visible among the essential workers were the uniformed first responders and health care professionals who worked directly with the sick and dying. Their heroism inspired daily cheers and handmade signs expressing thanks and support that appeared all around the city.

But their courage and commitment should not obscure the mistaken priorities, poor planning, and toxic inequalities that put them in mortal danger. The virus may have moved around the city at the speed of a cough, but the forces that undermined frontline workers were years in the making. A lack of basic medical supplies such as masks and protective gear, overcrowded housing that encouraged the spread of the virus, and inadequate health care messaging all exacerbated a grim situation. Television news coverage provided snapshots of dire conditions inside beleaguered hospitals, but for health care workers the surge in cases was a deadly crisis that they lived in for days on end. A report from the news service *Bloomberg* captured the painful inequality inscribed on the city, shaping conditions for health care workers and patients alike. From March to April 2020, cases in both Brooklyn and Queens surged to more than forty thousand. Brooklyn had only 2.2 hospital beds per 1,000 people, and Queens had 1.5 per thousand. Yet wealthier, whiter Manhattan had half as many cases and 6.4 hospital beds per 1,000 people.[1]

Confronted by a chaotic and rapidly evolving emergency, first responders and health care professionals were sustained by their commitment to their work, their professional training, and their loyalty to their co-workers. They were repeatedly forced to improvise solutions to urgent problems. Individual callings were reaffirmed and established hierarchies were upended.

In the grimmest days of the surge of 2020, New Yorkers leaned out their windows each night at 7:00 p.m. and cheered, clapped, banged pots, and played music to salute all the workers who faced death daily on their behalf. First responders and health care professionals had earned the daily cheers, but the ritual was about something more. In the nightly symphony, New Yorkers leaned out of their isolation to see and hear one another. Amid weeks of isolation and loneliness, each night their cheers let them know they were not alone.

"Dead on Arrival": A New York Fire Chief's
COVID-19 Journal

Simon Ressner

Simon Ressner, a 9/11 survivor, was a sixty-year-old battalion chief with the Fire Department of New York based in central Brooklyn at the start of the pandemic. He kept a diary of a twenty-four-hour shift that began at 9:00 a.m. on Friday, April 3, 2020. It was first published by ProPublica.[2]

"10–37 CODE 1."

It's fire department shorthand for "dead on arrival." Word of such tough calls crackles over the citywide radio in bursts.

One of my engines just returned from a 10–37 Code 1, and a firefighter is at my office door. He hands me what's called an "alarm ticket," and asks for a new supply of protective masks.

"Need four," he says, as if asking for some money for candy.

I ask about the run. "She had a fever, I reached out and touched her head and she was so hot."

I hand him four N95 masks, grab a disinfected pencil from my desk and mark on the inventory sheet: "Engine 235, Box location 431, Madison Street between Nostrand Avenue and Bedford Avenue."

It's around the corner from the firehouse, and so close that I can walk to my office's rear windows and see the building. Inside, an eighty-three-year-old woman with family nearby just died. Just outside my window.

While I'm attempting to get that to register, I hear several more 10–37 Code 1 signals come in. As I'm writing this, yet another one. The tone of the officer on the radio reporting the signal is matter of fact—not detached, more along the lines of, "Yep, another one."

10–37 Code 1. Another one a minute later.

I begin my shift at 9:00 a.m. I grab the bleach wipe from the canister, wipe down the computer keyboard, mouse, phone, desk and twenty other places where I can imagine anyone has put their hands.

I am working as chief in Battalion 57 of the FDNY, located in Bedford-Stuyvesant, Brooklyn. Bed-Stuy is a historically African American neighborhood that saw its population grow during the time when huge numbers of Southern Blacks migrated north, leaving agriculture work for ostensibly better jobs. In the last few years, it has undergone major gentrification, but it still remains culturally and demographically an African American neighborhood with a history of both hard times and cultural richness. Since almost all the country's past traumas have always hit the poor neighborhoods worst, I wonder what this worst situation, COVID-19, is going to entail and for how long.

I was a fireman here twenty-five years ago and now have returned as chief toward the end of my career. I thought that surviving September 11, 2001, would be the part of history I would tell grandchildren, but COVID-19 has clearly surmounted even that disastrous and heartbreaking day. The department lost 343; at least 50 of them were people I knew, including my chief, Dennis Cross. He taught me how to fight fires, but also how to sail a boat, and after his death his widow gave me use of his twenty-five-foot Catalina.[3]

I am focused on my work of supervising the four engine companies and two ladder companies of the 57, but I also have a ritual of checking the numbers: New York City Department of Health daily statistics; the Johns Hopkins website for worldwide information on COVID-19 cases and deaths. I quickly calculate the death percentages, taking comfort when I find the rate under 2 percent somewhere. But this morning the world figures show a rate of 5.23 percent, so I try and convince myself that it will drop because of the anomalies of Italy and Spain.

But the truth is that it is here in the United States where the percentages are climbing, and here in New York City where the numbers are headed toward the unfathomable. Every day I read the obituaries in the *New York Times* to remind myself of the pain that the families endure in a way that calculating the percentages can't. But I am waiting. I want to see those bars in the graphs get dramatically shorter.

Yesterday, I was tasked with approving hospital and nursing home requests to use the streets around their buildings to construct tents for overflow patients. Around 11:00 a.m., I received the first request of several to use the streets for refrigerated trailers to store the accumulating bodies. In the moment, I can be detached enough to do the work of looking at street dimensions, trailer sizes, locations of hydrants, and entrances to buildings in order to make it work. It takes me five minutes to look at that information and email back, "FDNY has no objection." And then a few more requests for more trailers. "FDNY has no objection."

Simple as that, we have approved the refrigerated storage on public streets of someone's relative.

I spend a good part of Friday morning rebalancing staffing in the fire companies in the battalion as well as the 31st Battalion in downtown Brooklyn. Staffing has become a challenge because, as of this morning, there are 1,056 firefighters, 686 EMS workers, and 115 FDNY civilians suspected of COVID-19 infection; 241 Fire personnel, 74 EMS, and 23 civilians have been confirmed. Fire companies that normally have twenty people on their roster are down to eleven, and so we move people from companies that have fared better to those companies that are depleted. Even now, there is still a fair amount of tangled paperwork to deal with.

After, I head down to the Chief's vehicle and start the next disinfecting ritual. The firefighters assure me that it has been done, but they are young and I am not. And they clearly haven't grasped the genuine risk we are facing with each contact with each other and each response for fires and emergencies.

I try to transmit a "10–18" as fast as I can when engines or trucks are responding to a fire. That signal allows me to hold one engine company and one ladder company at the scene and relieve the remaining three or four companies and get them back to their houses. I do this to limit the amount of time the firefighters hang out with each other talking, catching up, all typically done elbow to elbow. The faster I get the "18" out, the quicker I can keep them separated.

The sirens speak

Around noon, I watch Governor Andrew Cuomo's daily briefing on my computer. I haven't yet had a fire call, but I can hear the ambulance sirens regularly. People ask how I can tell what kind of siren it is, and I realize that I have to think about that: it's the absence of the air horns (the blasting trumpetlike sound) of our trucks and the absence of the "rumbler" that the New York Police Department uses. I definitely can tell. Another siren off in the distance—no air horn, no rumbler. It's EMS.

When you work twenty-four-hour shifts, it's often easy to be confused about what day of the week it is. But with COVID-19, I realize that there is no rhythm for anyone anywhere. I stop myself when I ask my wife, "What's going on this weekend?" There is no weekend, no beginning of the week. What does TGIF mean anymore?

For my wife, Moy, the load is devastating. She is an accountant for an urban planning firm, and like all her colleagues has been working from home. It is her job to get everything needed for a new PPP (payroll protection plan). The faster they get the money the more likely her firm can survive. She does all this while caring for her ninety-one-year-old mother, who lives with us and suffers from advanced dementia.

In the aftermath of 9/11, she attended every funeral from my company, six in all. And in "normal" years, she has endured all of the isolation, fear, and hardship that a family member of an active-duty firefighter can deal with. I never imagined in our lifetime we would be facing what is essentially an international plague. As late as February, we still couldn't imagine a world where the streets of New York are empty during rush hour. Or a world where—years after having to worry about infections because of damage my lungs had suffered on 9/11—I would once again have fear that I could die *of a virus!* by going to work.

My nose starts itching. DON'T TOUCH YOUR FACE!!

Up until recently, the Fire Department was able to switch and swap shifts in a way that led to different people working together in a random but ordered way. But with the department's response to COVID-19, we were organized into four platoons—A, B, C, and D. Everyone in each group would work with the same people each time their letter came up on the calendar. The idea was that if there was a person positive for COVID-19 in one particular group, it would only affect that particular group as opposed to infecting everyone in the company.

At the beginning of the outbreak, if someone tested positive and had been in close contact with other members, those members were directed to quarantine. Quickly that changed since the number of people testing positive was increasing rapidly. Within a week, the department revised the protocols and directed that members who were in contact with a suspected or known positive colleague should continue to work unless they exhibited symptoms. If symptoms came on, they would be placed on medical leave. During the "earlier" days of the pandemic, we all believed that you were only contagious if you had symptoms. And although we now know that is not the case, the manpower needs are such that without positive testing we continue to work until we have symptoms or if we have prolonged close contact with someone who has a positive test.

The interim lifesavers

The Fire Department started taking on medical calls in 1995 in order to help improve response time to serious medical emergencies by providing lifesaving care from a fire crew while awaiting transport and more advanced medical care by EMS. As a result, all firefighters are trained to provide some degree of emergency medical care, including the use of a defibrillator. But several hundred current firefighters are former EMS personnel who had transferred to the fire protection side of the department. With the number of COVID-19 cases accelerating daily, some of those more highly trained firefighters have been brought back to supplement EMS.

On medical runs, the firefighter's role is to provide patient evaluation, basic life support and first aid, and if needed perform CPR until better trained help arrives. They wear protective gloves, and administer only what's called BVM resuscitation efforts: bag, valve, mask, basically hand compressions and a device to get oxygen into lungs. Fire companies do not transport people to the hospital.

Those lifesaving protocols were shifted approximately a week ago. We always attempt to revive a patient and perform CPR, and still do. But now, our efforts are limited to twenty minutes, and so if there is no spontaneous pulse or defibrillation is unsuccessful, we cease. The exception is for what is called "obvious death," like rigor mortis, decomposition, dismemberment.

In the afternoon, I get a phone call from Fire Operations Command Center, "How many N95 masks you have in stock, Chief? We're doing the daily tally." I tell him the truth—84—and a cheerful voice says, "Great, you're in good shape then. Stay safe out there."

We all say it, we all mean it, but I know that it is, as the president would say, "aspirational." A month ago I was thinking about how to surprise my wife for our thirtieth anniversary. Perhaps San Francisco or London. How quaint. On April 7, my anniversary, I will return for my next twenty-four-hour shift.

Another siren: no air horn, no rumbler. EMS. Lunch is ready.

In emergency work, if your mind, or at least your behavior, can't adjust to what is actually happening and to deal with that as it is, you simply cannot help anyone. So the regular rhythm of 10–37 Code 1 mostly registers as a clear-eyed reminder of what is being confronted. Firefighters make this adjustment at lots of incidents: fires, car accidents, falls, construction accidents, and so on. But then there is a shift back to a world that is not tragic every day or even every week.

In 2019 there were sixty-six people who died in fires in all of New York City—in a year! So you deal with the fire, steel your emotions, revel in the action, recognize the loss, but then there is what seems to be a respite. I'm pretty sure that by the end of my twenty-four hours this shift, there will be at least sixty-six calls that I hear on the radio for COVID-19-related deaths.

Isn't there a quote about the banality of evil? The radio goes off again: "10–37."

At lunch, for all my desire to isolate from everyone, I stay longer than I should have because the laughter was soothing. Five young men, with some fear but mainly strength and youth on their psychological side.

Soon, the young firefighter who had got masks from me earlier was back. "I need four." I ask him if the patient was an elderly person. "Yes, and he was really thin," he tells me. I say that maybe it was a cancer patient, and sure enough, he hands me the dispatch ticket and right there it says, "Patient has Cancer."

My questions are in part meant to maintain my sense of empathy and in part to soothe my fear. I'll be okay even though I'm over sixty. I'll be okay because I don't have cancer.

"10–37 Code 1." I have truly lost count. At one point, while watching Norah O'Donnell's newscast, I hear several 10–37s. It feels like when it snows into your eyes, a little sting, a blink, a little sting.

The daunting curve

The message from New York State's health commissioner plays for the fiftieth time. Mild mannered, even bland, he espouses social distancing as if he's telling young kids to share their toys in the sandbox.

Returning from a fire run, we see a double-size city bus sailing down Nostrand Avenue. There are people seated throughout, and many sitting directly next to each other. That's one bus with twenty-five people who may infect forty who then may infect eighty more. I'm a trained engineer as well as a firefighter, and my mind pictures the exponential curve from math class: mercilessly steep and ever steeper over time.

When I got to Bedford-Stuyvesant more than two decades ago, it was considered a tough and dangerous place. And it was a tough and dangerous place. Murders were through the roof. But it was a place we all wanted to be. Everyone who worked here, in fact, had to know someone in order to be assigned—"a hook," someone who can pull a string or two.

Firefighters want to be where the action is, not because they are unfeeling or reckless but because we know that you can't be good at this without actually doing it. Over time, dealing with fires is something that combines art, science, and the deepest psycho-physiology of human performance under stress. It was exciting to be here in the nineties, it was a great place to learn this job, but I don't remember ever feeling this sense of looming menace. A dangerous neighborhood filled with beautiful brownstones, weary frame houses, and blocks and blocks of public housing is something your consciousness can quantify and manage. COVID-19 is too big and too dynamic. Even twenty-four-hour news can't give a sense of time passing. The numbers I saw before dinner were up by several hundred by the time I walked by the apple pie and went upstairs.

This isn't firefighting, this feels more like the crew on a sinking ship desperately trying to load the boats while the water gets ever closer.

I wish I had taken a piece of pie.

Into the Storm

Phil Suarez

Phil Suarez was born in France, has lived in Spain, and resides in Easton, Connecticut. A paramedic in New York City with more than twenty-five years of experience, for the past decade he has worked in Harlem and Washington Heights. He stayed at his job during COVID-19 despite its risks. "We're not special. We're not heroes. But this is our job. I couldn't live with myself if I abandoned my job in its most dire moment."[4]

I'VE ALWAYS WORKED in impoverished enclaves of New York City, immigrant communities.

As an immigrant I can relate to them better. I find them to be sometimes more real than more upscale areas like the Upper East Side where people may be more snobbyish or name dropping. I just find the underserved communities need the help. They need people that are probably a little more understanding of how they got there, what they may be going through. It probably comes from my background as an immigrant myself.

I've been doing this a long time. For me, it's a very easy job.

I'm drawn to it because an old partner of mine that's a writer said, "We knock on their doors, and they open their doors to us." For that half hour, we're an integral part of their crazy world, whatever that may be. And it's really crazy. It's almost like voyeurism. And it is addictive. Twenty plus years into this, I can still be stunned.

Most of our calls are very routine. And then you have your more chaotic scenes where there could be a trauma like a car accident, somebody stabbed, shot, for instance. You can go from doing nothing, from zero or five miles an hour to, all of a sudden, being like eighty miles an hour in this chaos. That's what our forte is. Most of us that have been doing this for a while, we kind of thrive in that chaos. I can't imagine working a controlled environment.

Preparing for the surge

I started preparing myself and with my supervisor we kind of took the reins. We started hoarding the PPE [personal protective equipment] as much as we could. Stashing it. People were kind of panicking and if they saw a roll of toilet paper, they would grab it. [*laughs*] If they saw N95s, they would grab them. So the hoarding became a problem 'cause you want to have stuff available for everybody.

I've worked many disasters and stuff like that. I was probably a little bit better prepared, and so saw that coming, I knew I would be good to the best of my abilities as far as PPE. That I would have enough for foreseeable future. And that's being diligent.

And all of a sudden, for the better part of three weeks, it seems like everything that we did was COVID-19. I think 98 percent of our call volume was all COVID-19 symptoms. All of a sudden it was before us. Came in very violent.

Everything I've done, I tried to take what I call a calculated risk. I was an avid mountain biker. I was a mountaineer, a rock climber, and stuff like that. So everything I did, I tried to do a calculated risk. How much risk am I taking here? Am I okay with it? What are my chances of really getting hurt?

I approached everything through my knowledge base. I told my supervisors and bosses I will keep coming to work as long as I have no fever, and I have a N95 to wear for the shift. The day I have a fever or I don't have an N95, I will not come to work. And that was my red line. There has to be a red line.

My personal feeling is that the health officials didn't take into consideration the risk that we were taking and the repercussions of those risks because we expose ourselves, we expose others.

Seeing EMTs without masks or without proper gear

I'm a paramedic. We're the highest level of care in prehospital. Then there's the EMTs that are basic. And often times, we back them up.

I was taking as many precautions as I could. And I would go into their ambulance and see that they had no mask on. I would pull them aside.

"Hey, where is your PPE?"

"Oh, no. No. He's got back pain."

I said, "No. He's got COVID-19. Back pain, mostly likely, is COVID-19."

At times, some of the EMTs or crew—some of the other crews that may have known better—I actually yelled at some of them. I would take them aside and just like, "What are you—you got to be smarter than this."

What was happening in March and April of 2020

We work in an immigrant community where there's six, eight people living in a small apartment. And some of these apartments we go in there, and you'd have half or three-quarters of the home exhibiting flulike symptoms, which most definitely were COVID-19. So we're not going to bring them to the hospital. There's risk of them infecting others. And health care workers. They're just going to be sent home. And was it ideal, looking back? Probably not. But it was what we had back then.

I carried a certain amount of guilt when we started realizing that some of these people that were having symptoms like low-grade temperature and mild shortness of breath within three days would go into the storm, and many ended up in life support or some of them succumbed to the virus.

But it's what we had on hand. It's what we knew. There was no alternative.

So I did my best to take my time in the homes and tell them about self-care. It seems that we have lost the ability to self-care over the years. Nobody has Tylenol anymore. Nobody knows to hydrate with water, not soda. Or to isolate yourself from the healthy.

I'd go into homes and the sick were sitting next to the healthy on the sofa. So that was kind of frustrating to see the public not doing their part, even the basics of self-care. And so I would tell them. Go take a shower. Hydrate. Eat good food. Build up your immune system. Stay away from fat and sugar and stuff like that. And drink a lot of water. Take Tylenol if you need to.

I made it a point to tell them to walk thirty feet. If they could walk thirty feet, just keep doing what they're doing. But once they can't walk a certain amount, you have to assume that they're desatting, that their oxygen saturation may be dropping. Then you need to be hospitalized. So I felt that was the best I could do with the information and the tools we had on hand.

People were scared to go to the hospital. As a matter of fact, I had to convince people to go to the hospital because they were so scared of COVID-19. I would tell them, "You most likely have COVID-19. So you're not going to recatch it. You have every symptom of coronavirus. You need to be hospitalized."

A day to remember

My worst day was April 6 or something like that. In one day, I had a fifteen-year-old, a twenty-five-year-old, a forty-two-year-old, and a fifty-six-year-old in cardiac arrest.

And they all died except for the twenty-five-year-old. The fifteen-year-old was difficult, but I knew she wasn't going to make it.

It was 6:00 a.m. I logged on to our computer in the ambulance and we get what's called a sprint, basically a transcription of the 9-1-1 call. And it says, "Fifteen-year-old, cardiac arrest, CPR in progress by family."

And I told the dispatcher, "You're reading the same thing as I'm reading. It's a child in cardiac arrest. Can you send me somebody? I'm coming from a distance. I'm coming from Manhattan."

And they're like, "You're solo. Do your best."

So we hauled over there to the Bronx. It's a fifth floor walkup. We load up fifty pounds of gear, go up five flights of stairs.

At that point, fire got there. And she was asystolic. [Her heart had stopped beating.] We tried to work her up. I was very aggressive, obviously. And the best we got was a PEA, a pulseless electrical activity, briefly. Then she went right back into asystolic.

I know there was nothing more I could have done. But it still—fifteen years old. Obviously, it weighs very heavily on anyone. And the family was there. It was just very, very traumatic. But the rest of the day didn't get any better.

And oddly enough, three of them that I had, they had the same scenario. They had these low symptoms. And they were about to go into the shower. And then they went into cardiac arrest. And all of a sudden they would just drop dead.

And this twenty-five-year-old was the same thing. It was bizarre. I don't know why.

The twenty-five-year-old, he had just gone down. I wanted to give him every chance possible, so I'm like, "You know what? I'm just going to do a endotracheal intubation" [insert a tube into his windpipe to deliver oxygen], which is riskier obviously. And we worked him up for about fifteen minutes and got him back.

How he did, I don't know. It was just too many patients to follow up on. But I think it was pretty promising. But I, unfortunately, don't know his final outcome. I hope it was good. I told myself that it was maybe good.

So that was my worst day. I was averaging about three cardiac arrests a shift, which is unprecedented. That day was four, but that day made it worse. Just the ages. It was such young people. And that just puts a lot into perspective. It's so frustrating to read and to hear what we hear knowing what we saw and witnessed.

Being in harm's way

With COVID-19, I have to say, at first, I think I was going to get it, and I was likely going to die. And that was scary. I think that's probably what caused a lot of anxiety. All these people are getting it. I'm not special. [*laughs*] And I'm a male. I'm well into my forties. I'm probably going to get it. And I'm going to die. Or be really messed up from it. And that was hard. That was one of the hardest things I've probably had to personally dwell with in my life.

I talked about it with my wife. Talked about it with myself a lot. And I just kind of liked my job. I know some people kind of stopped working because the risk was too much.

We're not special. We're not heroes. But this is our job. I couldn't live with myself if I abandoned my job in its most dire moment. It's what we chose to do. For better, for worse, we mitigate the risk, and we try to do our job. And that was what I told myself.

At the end of my shift, I would get in my car. I would take a bottle of Purell and literally rub it all over my face, shove it up my nose, in my ears, my hair. For the first week or so, we had Lysol, so we would spray ourselves down with Lysol. And if it was on us, at least try to kill it before you go home.

I would drive home for about an hour. Sometimes I would find myself with my mouth gaping open just staring. Just kind of trying to process what the last eight, sixteen hours have been like. It's truly a profound moment.

I would get home, go in the garage, strip down to my birthday suit. My wife would be out there with a garbage bag, put all my stuff in there, then she would take the clothes, put it in the washing machine. And I would go into the shower and literally loofah five layers of skin off of me. I mean literally clawing my skin off to hopefully get rid of the stuff.

Anxiety

I had a huge amount of anxiety, which is something I've never really experienced before.

I wasn't sleeping much. I was constantly thirsty. I was barely eating. I had no appetite. I was so thirsty. I could not drink enough water in a shift. And thereafter, when I was reading stuff, I started realizing these are all signs of anxiety. These are all signs of stress.

I tried to come home and decompress. Kind of just shut that out. I stopped reading a lot of media stuff, especially social media. That I avoided like a plague itself. I read just headlines. And then when I would come home, I would make it a point that with the family just try to talk about COVID-19 or get it out of your system. Talk about it. And then talk [*laughs*] about something else. But it was difficult. It dominated our whole lives for that time. It really did. I'm sure I'm not alone in this.

Sources of information

We had nothing. [*laughs*] And even if we did, I would take that with a grain of salt. It's like reading the news nowadays. You really have to dig around five, six sources. I double check my sources.

I only read what I feel are trusted sources and try to just drown out all the misinformation that is so prevalent [*laughs*] and so toxic. We really don't get [*laughs*] memos, meetings. Nothing. It's incredible but not surprising. [*laughs*]

Did the city provide services or debriefings?

No. No. No. [*laughs*] No. I had no expectations of it either. We never have. [*laughs*] As like 9/11. Just get back to work. [*laughs*] Sometimes—I always felt that that's one of the bad things of our profession. There's no sort of like decompression like somebody steps in.

But I do feel that it should be there for the psychological well-being of anybody, whether it's a social worker, a doctor, nurse, whoever. We're human after all. We have to process this stuff.

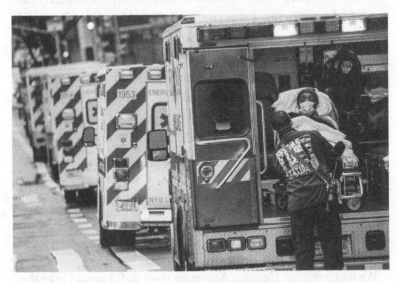

FIGURE 4
April 13, 2020: ambulance crew and patient outside NYU Langone Hospital in Manhattan. Photograph by John Minchillo, Associated Press.

Challenging Times

Richard Brea

Richard Brea, commander of the 46th Precinct in the Bronx when COVID-19 struck, is the son of immigrants from the Dominican Republic. Brea was born in Queens and raised there in Richmond Hill, where his father was a cook and his mother was a seamstress. Brea became a police officer in 1993 at twenty-one and worked in Brooklyn, the Bronx, and Manhattan on patrol, special operations units, and on assignments ranging from narcotics to anticrime. He rose through the ranks to become a deputy inspector and precinct commander.[5]

THE MORE WE started learning about it, how COVID-19 was spreading, and how other countries were having challenges with it, more people started getting concerned about it.

Working in the New York City Police Department presented a challenge for us. Other employers allowed their employees to work remotely; we couldn't do that.

Officers had to answer calls in apartments where people had died of COVID-19.

Some officers were concerned about their safety responding to a call where somebody's coughing and fearing that they might be infected. They were also taking people to hospitals where there was a high rate of positive cases and posed a significant risk of transmission, which concerned many officers.

For those officers who were deeply concerned about COVID-19 exposure, I told them: "Unfortunately, this is no different than responding to an active shooter scenario, or somebody shooting a gun." We must respond to these calls, that's our profession, that's what we chose to do. And we did. It was challenging, but we responded to these calls.

And I think most officers understood that and accepted it as another hazard of the job. It was like responding to a gun run, or a burglary in progress. It was dangerous, but they did it.

We accepted the dangers when we raised our hands and swore an oath to become police officers.

I told them you've got to do the best you can to protect yourself—wear masks.

The New York City Police Department and the city of New York supplied us with the equipment we needed at the time such as masks, gloves, and hand sanitizers. The response was fairly quick, and the supply was constant.

Some cops felt that we were very exposed to this virus. And we probably were. We saw a sharp increase in DOAs, dead persons in apartments. On a particular tour, we could have four or five deaths that were most likely the result of COVID-19.

Some officers were concerned. "Why is it safe for us to go into the apartment?" And I said, I understand that, and I understand your concern.

I went to some of these apartments with the officers so that they knew we were facing these challenges together.

It was a tough time, because anytime you deal with a death, it's very emotional for the family.

But many of these deaths were untimely in the sense that, although many of them were elderly and suffered from other illnesses, these deaths were occurring virtually overnight. And that was shocking for many family members.

And sometimes people would die alone in their apartment because the family wouldn't be able to travel. And sometimes the families were also concerned: If this person passed away from COVID-19, is it safe for me to go there?

There were a lot of unknowns at the time. How is this being transmitted? Early on, there were many different rumors.

So, my concern was, how is exactly is this virus transmitted, and there seemed to be, at the time, conflicting opinions about it.

There was a lot of anxiety because of that. There were a lot of things that made people upset because nobody really knew. And it was a tough position for the doctors and scientists —which is understandable for me. I'm not a doctor. I'm not a scientist. But I listen.

My focus was to reassure my officers that we had a job to do, and that we should use every precaution that we could to protect ourselves by utilizing the masks and hand sanitizers, which is what we were told at the time, the most effective way to combat this virus. My civilian cleaners in the precinct did a tremendous job of constantly cleaning all the hard surfaces to minimize exposure.

It was challenging when more of my officers began testing positive with COVID-19. Suddenly, our positive COVID-19 rate increased significantly. And that was very, very concerning for everyone. Especially for me, since I am responsible to ensure the safety of my officers.

The department kept track of positive COVID-19 status. And the 46th Precinct at the time had one of the highest rates of positive exposures.

Brea contacted officers who got sick.

I would call my officers frequently, to see how they were doing. Some of them I called two or three times a week.

Their symptoms varied a lot. Some officers had no symptoms. But other officers had some very severe symptoms, and I could hear them on the phone. And these were young officers. Some of them had difficulty speaking, they were coughing a lot. And they really sounded bad.

One of the officers that I spoke with was coughing a lot, could barely breathe, and had tremendous pain. It was so bad that I felt guilty even calling them because they were struggling just to talk.

And they gave me permission to relay their stories to other officers, and I would. Because I felt that it was important that they knew that COVID-19 was very serious, and this was affecting all of us. I would inform the other officers to keep our sick officers in your thoughts and prayers. Many officers would respond to them via email or text with encouraging messages, lifting their spirits.

When I started doing that, I noticed more officers taking COVID-19 seriously. It wasn't just people in the street getting sick, we were getting sick, too. We have to do what we can to protect ourselves. That was part of my role as a precinct commander, to ensure that that the officers knew that this was serious and that they protected themselves.

I kept thinking to myself, wow, these are young officers. They're in the twenties, early thirties. They're having a tough time with this. I can only imagine if someone older like myself got it, how severe would the symptoms be?

Going home

For me, it was a challenge going home, and making sure that I didn't bring something home to my family as well.

One officer, his parents were elderly, and he didn't want to take that chance. They had a single-family home, and he would just stay in the basement. I felt bad for him since he didn't have any personal contact with them. But at least he was grateful that he could do that. Some people couldn't do that, they lived in small apartments and, unfortunately, going home meant you were exposing your loved ones.

I attempted to make some accommodations for officers who had difficult situations at home. One officer had an elderly mother who was very ill, and if she were to be exposed to COVID-19, it would probably be fatal. The officer was very scared that she would be exposed to COVID-19 at work and unknowingly bring it home to where they lived in a small apartment. So, I did what I could to try to limit her exposure in the field.

But unfortunately, you couldn't protect everyone. Police needed to be in the streets. Most officers didn't mind. Some of the younger officers thought that this virus was exaggerated, this wasn't a big deal.

Within the 46th Precinct, to reduce transmissions of COVID-19, Brea reorganized procedures like roll call, signing out at the end of a shift, signing out equipment, and cleaning cars.

At the time, I had to stress the importance of wearing masks to the officers. I wore a mask in order to lead by example. I couldn't tell someone else to wear a mask if I wasn't wearing one either. So, I would always wear my mask. And then I would ask my officers, "Hey, where's your mask?" And I always carried at least five masks with me. If an officer told me, "I don't have one," I would say, "Well, here you go, now you do."

As commander of the 33rd Precinct in southern Washington Heights, Brea learned the challenges and rewards of working with neighborhood residents to address issues ranging from the mentally ill homeless to gangs. He carried lessons learned in the 33rd Precinct to his Bronx command.

Early in the pandemic, street crime decreased because there were fewer people in the street. Unfortunately, we quickly started seeing an increase in other crimes such as burglaries because many establishments were closed, and bad people knew that. So, the stores started getting burglarized. Jewelry stores, pawn shops, sneaker stores, and even restaurants were hit. Then unfortunately, as more people worked from home, we started seeing an increase in domestic violence cases.

Brea knew of police officers elsewhere in the New York City Police Department who died of COVID-19, but under his command the 46th Precinct did not lose any officers to COVID-19.

On the Frontlines of COVID-19, Echoes of AIDS

Steven Palmer

Steven Palmer is a physician assistant and clinical coordinator of the HIV vaccines unit who works with other clinicians and research assistants at Columbia University Medical Center. All were redeployed full time to treat COVID-19 in the surge of spring 2020.[6]

I DON'T THINK I could have ever prepared for what the surge was going to be like. I heard about what was happening in Italy, but it was . . . Oh, God. My metaphor is we were like a bunch of ants standing on our back legs with our front legs in the air and a meteor is coming. And it was frightening. It was FRIGHTENING!

People have told me that I'm on the frontlines, and I want to show lots of deference to people who are on the fronter frontlines. The clinicians, the EMTs, the patient reps, anybody who was in the emergency room, anybody who was in the ICUs, I just want it known that they were the front-front-front-frontlines. Frontlines is a spectrum and I'm now willing to accept that I was on the frontlines, given some retrospect, but those folks were right there.

Palmer reviewed patients' charts, drew blood from patients, monitored their treatment, and asked their permission to try an experimental treatment for COVID-19. When a patient was unable to give their consent because they were intubated, he sought permission from family members. One day, in the early weeks of the pandemic, when cases were increasing, he entered an ICU in the Allen Hospital in the Inwood section of northern Manhattan.

I noticed one nurse in front of her computer. She was very, very nice and very helpful. But she started mumbling to herself a little bit like, "How are we going to do this without getting infected?"

The folks who were right there, the vision that they had wasn't that 99 percent were going to be better. It was that you were going to be intubated, and that there was a good chance you might die.

And I still have to try to get that out of my head sometimes. You know? If I feel a little warm when I'm walking in the woods or something, you know, I'm like, oh geez. I better go take my temperature when I get back.

Conditions at the Harkness Pavilion in Washington Heights, site of his office

The patients were starting to take up the ICUs and then they had to convert the ORs into ICUs as well. And then the floor above me, the research floor, became COVID-19 patients only so the numbers started piling up. The oncology department people were redeployed. People who had worked in otolaryngology were now in ICUs and scared to death. They don't know what they're doing. It's like being an oral historian and now you're a cobbler, except that's less scary.

There were many things that were disturbing. First is that the Harkness Pavilion, lots of the floors were vacated. People went home and did telemedicine. So, there was also a feeling of eeriness of all of these hallways with nobody in them. And then the oncology nurses were redeployed to us and started working with us. They were redeployed to us and they were *great*. They're young. They're nimble. They understand technology, all of this, in a way that I just never will and were able to help organize things for us in terms of entering data on patients and that made our lives immeasurably better.

Across the street is the Milstein building and on the second floor is a catwalk from one building to the other. I look out and I recognize that at the side of the Milstein building are two large refrigerator trucks and that's where the bodies are going. There's a tent set up before it and then there's these two trucks and I just knew that they were just being filled.

Back to the OR ICU for one moment. It was my turn to go in there, and it's when it was at its height and there were five operating rooms side by side and each one had people intubated. It was like walking into a horror movie. You walked in there, and I just felt like I'm a goner.

Every time I passed hand sanitizer, I put my hand under it. I probably cleaned my hands fifty, sixty times a day and that's not an exaggeration. At first, I was going over with gloves on, and it became clear to me after a while that gloves give you the impression that you're clean. You're not remembering that you've contaminated them all along the way and then you're touching something that somebody else may touch and then rub their nose because they weren't thinking about it.

For Palmer, the COVID-19 pandemic brought up memories of the AIDS epidemic.

In early March, a friend and I went to a restaurant the last days before they closed. And I knew something was coming but I didn't know it was going to crush us. I had no idea. And he said, "Steven, does this remind you of AIDS at all, your experience of the eighties?" And I kind of brushed it off. I was just like, "You know, I don't think so. This is very contagious." He was much more astute than I was. And over time, these parallelisms started happening. The reason I recognized them is because they came up emotionally.

I'm up in Liberty, New York, right now. The Woodstock site is fifteen minutes away. And I just felt like I needed some space. It's a beautiful place, and I was there one day and there was a young guy probably in his mid-late twenties and he was just visiting also. He had in the last couple of years spread his mom and his grandfather's ashes on the field. We were chatting and I'm noticing, you know, even though we're talking forward that we're like only two feet away from each other. I was like, "Oh geez, you know, what am I doing here?" Then I made it three feet and I'm thinking, "Well, you should make it six feet." And then I thought, "Oh, he's a handsome young man. Look at him. He's very nice and engageable."

And then it was time for me to leave and I got in my car and I felt like it had been 1986 and I had had drunken, wanton sex and did I use a condom?

What allowed me to not take care of myself? Was I taking care of myself? Maybe I was. I was like, holy crap. This is almost like the same feeling. And that's when it occurred to me that there were parallels and that maybe other people had felt that too.

Visiting his partner requires precaution that recall the AIDS years.

We generally use a different bathroom. We sleep in different beds. So, it takes a toll. There's an emotional toll to this to being on the frontlines, wherever I am on that spectrum.

As we lighten up about the pandemic, we're reminded at times that it's not over by any stretch of the imagination and we could still be exposed. And what does that mean for those of us who are working in this field? How are we able to be with others around us and how long can we put up with that for?

On top of everything we're feeling, we're not supposed to be near anybody. It's a terrible combination. The first three weeks were terrible. I'd wake up and the first thing that came to my mind was coronavirus. I would actually have to talk to a friend of mine to help bolster myself. I was sobbing almost every morning.

With therapy, Palmer figured out that part of what he was experiencing during COVID-19 was post-traumatic stress from the AIDS years.

I was able, to some extent, to compartmentalize that this is an old thing—this overlap with HIV, and then gradually over time it took its kind of rightful place in my own emotional history. And then I was just dealing with what was right in front of me and was able to get past this parallel experience with HIV in the 1980s.

It was helpful for me to figure it out because it made me recognize a way in which I was going to be able to deal emotionally with what was coming up. There was a precedent to it, and I had the help I needed to move on. The early days of HIV became a reference point – something I could relate to quite concretely rather than just being in this nightmarish cosmic blur of bodies piling up, and you have to run over there quick to help out, and the wind is blowing at you from the OR, and you're feeling grief. We had been here before in some form or fashion, and that helped me think about how we'd get through this too.

About two and a half weeks ago I heard that only 500 had died, which is awful for every one of those people and everybody grieving around them. So, this odd split of being like, oh wow, only 500. Oh, now we're down to only 450. And being glad about that, you know, that it's not 800 anymore. It's a weird split when you're in the momentum of this kind of thing.

Coping strategies outside of work

I walk a lot. I try to walk every day up to Fort Tryon Park. Springtime, the Heather Gardens up at Fort Tryon Park, that kind of beauty, verdant beauty, green coming in, that helps.

Since January 2018 I've started taking Fridays off, so I have three-day weekends. I was working five days a week when the surge started because that's how it had to happen. I'm back to four days until future notice and I take lots of walks in nature. Nature really helps. A friend who is a yoga instructor is giving free thirty-minutes to essential workers, and I've used that a few times and that has been very helpful. Having therapy. Saying to myself that I can quit this if I want to at a certain point, knowing that I won't. That would sit terribly on me but just reminding myself that there's a way out.

And there's one other aspect. It's a little new-agey if you don't mind. The therapist I work with does EMDR [eye movement desensitization and reprocessing] and for years and years she brought people to Peru on shamanic journeys. It's the reminder to myself that the warrior spirit is in place and it's moving forward. And even though when the surge first came, my images of me were me crumbling—seriously just crumbling, like I was one of the ants with my hands in the air—this plays a role at least to me as an initiation rite into the next chapter of my life. And there's kind of a scarification aspect of it, but that I will emerge and it'll be okay, and that in some ways things that seemed important, or scary, or worrisome to me earlier will take their place of being, "so what?" That's the hope. It's a vision I have of how this can work itself through with me.

I'm going back to the city tonight. It does help to have that perspective in place because these things do subside even if we think it's never going to. In a grander spiritual vision, I wish humanity would change. We're the only species who doesn't live in symbiosis with the earth. We come in and we command that it conform to us.

I wish mother nature wouldn't have to take a breath just to deal with us. And she unleashes. And I just hope we don't miss this moment.

I'm going to take the dog for a nice long walk. The birds are singing. It's a beautiful—it's almost like sixty-five degrees out right now. I'll absorb nature as much as I can so that I can go back there and put up with it for four days or whatever.

At the Gates of Hell

Patricia Tiu

Patricia Tiu, a nurse, is the daughter of immigrants from the Philippines and a lifelong resident of Queens who lives in Fresh Meadows. She was working at New York–Presbyterian/Weill Cornell Medical Center in Washington Heights when the pandemic hit; she recorded her observations in video journals that were posted online.[7]

MARCH 29, 2020

Even though I understand the severity of this virus, I underestimated the impact it would have on the American health care system, for damn sure. I never thought it would get to the point that it is now. It shouldn't have ever gotten to this point. Everyone needs to know what exactly is happening, because it's not going to end well.

The week that just passed we officially all went to the ICU and no longer the ER because the ER, they're flooded. The hospital made every single nurse step up from what they usually are doing. Nurses have to become full blown ICU nurses. And to become a full blown ICU nurse you usually need at least very minimum six months orientation. All of a sudden, a week. It's like throwing a golfer to go play basketball, in a week they should learn and compete in the NBA.

The FDA was saying because we're so short of supplies, if you have a patient with the same disease, it's okay to use the same pair of gloves which is disgusting. The N95s: we were given one and they said keep it for a week.

I just want to give you a heads up of what it means to be on a ventilator. You need a vent because your lungs get so filled with fluid you're drowning in your lungs.

The biggest part has been getting people off the vents. When you're on a vent, it's usually maybe two or three days depending on how sick you are. When you're on a vent as a COVID-19 patient, your minimum is two weeks. We've had patients on it for a month.

Cuomo has been begging for vents. And you know that the whole thing was the supplies. And then Trump was saying that New York City is exaggerating the amount of vents we need. I really hope so because pretty soon you are going to have to choose who gets vented and who doesn't get vented. And what that entails is basically who gets to live and who doesn't get to live. Does your sixty-five-year-old grandma get to live or your forty-year-old neighbor?

As an American, born and raised in Queens, it is a fucking shame that our government can't get us the supplies that we need. You can't say we don't have the resources. This is not oil that we're fucking asking for. This is things that we can find and make on our soil, and it's absolutely disgusting how they just show that they don't give a fuck about us. Not just the nurses and the health care staff just us in general, like the majority, the working class. And they made that very apparent.

So what does it mean to be a COVID-19 positive patient that's on a vent? It means that you're in the room alone. And when we come in and care for you, we're not trying to be in there long. You're paralyzed. You're sleeping. I don't know if you hear us maybe you can, maybe you can't. But you're just there.

And as for our COVID-19 patients if you die, you die alone. Your family never gets to see you again. Not at least while you're breathing. You can't say goodbye; you can't even see what's happening.

Here's an example. And it's going to be a lot to hear.

There was an eighteen-year-old that was positive and vented, and I don't know what the full story was, but became brain dead.

So the doctors need the vent. So they called his mother. They explained that we got to pull the plug. Mother said, "Please no don't pull the plug just put the phone next to him. He will hear me and he'll wake up."

Like where does that put all of us? Where does that put every single person, the doctors, the mother, the eighteen-year-old, the staff, the person who's going to need the vent? Like what do you say to that? How would you handle that? What decision would you make? What if there was another eighteen-year-old who needs that vent? What are you supposed to do?

I don't know what you do with a situation like that. And if we run out of vents, that's what's going to happen. You're going to pick and choose. We have no choice but to see who would survive.

One of the patients had surgery. I forgot what she had, but she wasn't the healthiest person. I think maybe she had some sort of cancer. She's in the hospital now for like a week.

Then she just progressively didn't do well. She came into the hospital negative. She is now positive. She had to get intubated. She did not want to get intubated.

The last word she was saying is "I don't want to die alone." She asked the nurse if the nurse could stand where she could see her until she falls asleep from the sedation because she doesn't want to die alone. That was the last thing she said. [*Gets emotional*] So that's just like a hint of what's been going on.

Our own staff got hit. We have two doctors and a nurse as well are intubated and they're COVID-19 positive.

As for nurses: None of us are sleeping. I don't sleep anymore. Everybody has that high anxiety deep in them. Although I'm proud of our nurses, they're functioning and they're fighting through, that high anxiety twenty-four hours a day, seven days a week is killer.

We are not expendable. So all my nurses if you do not get the proper gear, your life is not worth losing. You deserve to come home to a family too.

April 6, 2020

I'm wearing a bandana not to look cute, but because of all the stress, my hair has started to fall out, which is not the worst thing in the world. It's hair. I'll grow back. But it's just really annoying.

I am now in hospital housing, which is basically a hotel. It was nice of them to offer, but I don't got a microwave here. I don't have any amenities. So I made the best of it.

The last time I spoke, I said New York City was on fire. Well, welcome to hell. Because we are basically at the gates of hell. We are very close from the tipping point, reaching the peak, we're almost there. We haven't reached it yet.

I have accepted the fact that our government, our president, and no one is coming to help. So New York, it's just us. No one is coming to help us. And working in this ICU, the number-one goal is basically to save as many lives as possible. Everybody's dying, and you're just doing your best to keep every single one of these people alive. Every minute that I have gone into work, you are working at like 150 percent. You don't even have time to think your own thoughts. You do everything, everything you can to make sure they're breathing.

The one thing I really feel is anger. And I'm angry. We are in war. You know New York is in war when we're by ourselves. And I've accepted that. But I'm never going to forget anything that's happened here.

The nurses are being spread so thin, so thin. What they're asking for us to do is beyond God's work. We're going to keep fighting, it's our city. So just keep spreading awareness, stay inside.

I stepped out today to do some groceries and errands and it's amazing to me how many people are still outside walking around even with no mask acting like nothing happened. I just I don't understand. And we are not at the worst yet. These next two weeks are going to be brutal. Like brutal. I'm telling you. [*sighs*] And no one is coming. No one is coming to help us. So for all my nurses hang in there. Stay strong. Have each other's back.

Don't be afraid. This is a very scary situation. It's a very anxious situation. Be smart about things but don't be afraid; if anything, be angry and let that anger fight because I'm angry.

In an interview with Jamie Beckenstein of the Queens Memory Project in June 2020, she recalled the hardships of the first stage in the pandemic.

I think one of the toughest moments for me was preparing this one patient to see his daughters. This was a single father who might have been in his fifties who had two daughters. I think one might have been my age and the other one was like twenty years old. And from the background history that I got, their mom might have passed away a while ago. It was just them three, there was no other family.

Preparing the room for them to see their father, I had to make a barrier between him and another patient that was in the room so they can have privacy. So we got two IV poles and tied a sheet and put it in between them. Just so the family members could have privacy and tell their dad that they love him.

God forbid, what would you do if this was your father that you had to say goodbye to with a tube down the throat, their eyes closed? And as I put it up, I remember walking out the room feeling very defeated.

But you just have to keep going. You shake it off, walk out, get your one minute of emotion that you're allowed to feel and go straight back to work. I think that might have been one of the hardest things I've ever done in my life.

It Was Not Business as Usual

Christopher Tedeschi

Christopher Tedeschi, an emergency physician, works at the Columbia Medical Center and the Allen Hospital in northern Manhattan, where he has additional responsibilities for teaching and operational planning. A lover of the outdoors, he focuses his work on disaster medicine and wilderness medicine. At the start of the pandemic, he was living in Harlem with his wife, Kiran, who is also an emergency physician at the Medical Center, and their two daughters. He was one of several people responsible for managing the response in the Medical Center emergency department.[8]

WE RAMPED UP things really, really quickly because the number of patients was enormous. We were overwhelmed in many ways.

The last week in March was the week where we saw the most patients in the ER. We were seeing more than two hundred patients per day in the ER on 168th Street, just for COVID-19. No one came to the ER for anything else. We were joking for a month that "nobody's had appendicitis in Manhattan." We still don't know what happened to them, or had a heart attack or a stroke, for that matter.

The single memory I'll take with me clinically is of the Allen Hospital, our smaller hospital. It's on 220th Street and Broadway, Manhattan. It serves Inwood and Riverdale and part of the South Bronx, that's where one of the highest concentrations of cases were.

Everyone always refers to the ER as "organized chaos," or something tacky like that. But for the most part, things are not out of control. It's an emergency department. It's meant for emergencies. People get shot. That's what we're there for.

When it becomes overwhelming, not only are you sailing through a storm, but you're not steering the boat, you're just hoping the boat doesn't tip over. In that hospital, we got to that point. And when I look back on it, I just see myself in the middle of that ER in the middle of the night making sure people's oxygen didn't run out. And it did. And that was not business as usual.

Lorna Breen, director of the Allen Hospital Emergency Department, contracted COVID-19 in March 2020. On April 26, she took her own life.

That lack of being able to steer the ship, to my mind, contributed greatly to Lorna taking her life. I don't know much more about her psyche than you'll read in the newspaper, but she was interested in being in control of her environment. And when that's taken away from you, it's very unsettling.

In their responses to COVID-19, doctors and hospital staff combined planned responses and improvisation.

We have a pretty robust preparedness. Not to speak the party line, but we did pretty well. Were we prepared for this one? Not entirely. Absolutely not. Should we have been? This is a once in a lifetime event. A lot of improvisation went on.

The biggest problem was, there was not enough nurses. It's as simple as that.

And what was even more unsteadying was that we were improvising medically. It's not like this was a disease we knew much about. We intubated so many people, put them on mechanical ventilators in the beginning. We learned over weeks that we probably didn't need to, and that was probably not the best thing. But we learned that from going through it.

Medically, we'll be on a little bit better footing next time. But that's unsettling to a bunch of physicians who, not only do they not have the stretchers to put the patients in, but they're not so sure even what to do with the patient once they're in the stretcher.

The biggest challenge that Tedeschi faced

The thing that is still hardest is that it comes home with you. I worked in Puerto Rico after Maria, I worked in Haiti after the earthquake. I worked after Sandy, but none of those things come home with you. None of those things come home to your two kids not going to school.

The other thing that was additionally energy consuming was having this group of people that we work with filter lots of needs and questions and concerns and anxieties. One of my jobs during all of this was doing the point person for communicating with our group. So I was the one that was sending the email every night, and I was the one who was answering people's questions and picking up the phone.

There were a lot of unanswerable questions, and a lot of anxiety. It's one of those situations where the uncertainty was really high, because no one knew what was going on. And the real risk and the perceived risk were really high, too; 25 percent of our nurses and beyond were out sick. Two of our staff members in the ER died of COVID-19.

So, the risk is real. Especially at the beginning. Everyone that got it, got it in those first few weeks because we were looking for people who had traveled from China and the cat was out of the bag, long before that.

I remember somebody saying, "Unless you see the person get hit by the car in front of you, and that's why they're in the ER, just assume they have COVID-19." And then, it became, "Even if they get hit by a car and they come into the ER, just assume they have it anyhow." And once we got to that point, seeing your colleagues get sick didn't happen as much.

Oftentimes with a big event, you can wake up the next morning and you can say, "It's over." 9/11, the next day it was horrible, but it was over.

I think one of the things that lots of people are struggling with are, we still wear our masks all day every day. We still have COVID-19 patients in the ER and we're not going to wake up one particular morning and brush ourselves off and say, "That's over now." That makes it hard.

Established hierarchies and improvisation in the emergency room

Our hospital system to begin with is very hierarchical, top-down, although it seems like 90 percent of the people are in middle management. The verdict comes from the top, so to speak. But there were definitely points where big gaps got exposed.

We encountered a lot of situations that we hadn't encountered before. The example that has come up in that regard was, again, at the Allen. The Allen ER has about twenty-four beds. And one night, when there were seventy-something patients there, it became clear that these people needed to go somewhere. But there was not one person who had the knowledge and power and authority and responsibility to make that happen. So that's where the organizational improvisation came in.

Sometimes it worked, and sometimes it didn't. That night, it worked because one of the administrators in our group just made it happen. We got a bunch of people transferred from one hospital to another. But I think that if you were to talk to a lot of more frontline types, you might find a lot of different opinions as to how well it was organized or how it was organized.

The problem at the Allen was, we had nowhere to put these critically ill patients. There are obviously other spaces to expand into. One of those spaces was the place where they do minor surgeries, like ambulatory surgeries. That was converted into an ICU, and it was great. They did it overnight, they put these air filters in. It just worked out. It was nice.

It was an enormous effort on the part of the hospital, and you can't create staff and nurses out of thin air. So, I don't think we could have been much more prepared. I think that there's a psychological thing that clicks that enables you to say, "Oh boy, we better turn this unit into an ICU." There's a hump to get over and you've got to jump. And we did. We did, for the most part.

In emergency rooms, doctors and nurses typically confront problems that are open to an immediate solution. Facing COVID-19, they were forced to provide palliative care that eased patients' suffering without being able to provide an immediate solution to their illness.

We experienced palliative care in the ER in a way that we never had before because so many people were sick and so many people were there for days, even more than usual. Our nurses did things during those few weeks that they don't do, from the technical ICU type stuff to turning off the ventilator on people. That's not part of our normal thing. We're not wholesale, not dozens of people at a time.

Last words

There's a tablet and a family member who doesn't know what's going on and an interpreter because they're not speaking the same language as you. There's all these layers between you and the person you're trying to talk to. And what you're trying to say is, "Your loved one's not going to survive." That's not day-to-day ER nursing or doctoring. But a lot of that happened.

Looking back on the pandemic in late March and early April of 2020

We're so lucky that this wave has passed us, and we can certainly look back analytically and figure out what we did wrong and what we need to do next time and all that. But also, I'm realizing how it was very consuming. I didn't exercise. I put on weight. I put everything aside. Everything stopped. We lost some co-workers. The impact of all of that is a little clearer now. People asked me throughout this, "How are you doing? How are you doing?"

And I would routinely say to them, "Ask me in six weeks." And luckily, here we are, six weeks later and I think that, looking back, you can see the bigness of it from the perspective of spending time in an ER.

I look at my kids. The impact has been enormous. My daughter Lena, she was in first grade. The last day she went to school was in the middle of March and thank God her closest companion is her four-year-old sister. That's an enormous impact on a seven-year-old. She didn't see her friends, she didn't go to school.

We have learned a lot, and we have learned our lesson, to some degree. But it's not fun.

Where the system failed

Well it's political, right? It failed in communication. It failed in messaging. But on the deeper level, it's a little bit about just compassion. There was a quote in the paper today from a twenty-something-year-old who isn't wearing a mask somewhere: "Well if I get the virus, God forgive me. I'm not going to stop my life for some virus." While I see where someone's coming from— the messaging and the communication has been so inconsistent and horrible, and the leadership on the national level has been so counterproductive, it's criminal—compassion is this desire to avoid suffering, prevent suffering, or relieve suffering. I don't know that that guy interviewed in the paper was coming from a place of being motivated to relieve suffering or thinking about relieving someone's suffering. That's the story of the last several years of our American culture to some degree.

From a political standpoint and from a health security policy standpoint, we've made a lot of bad decisions over the last five years, which is too bad. But frankly, I can't say I'm surprised at the outcome. When you take the system apart, the system doesn't work. And to some degree, we took the system apart. And to hear the political rhetoric, the politically motivated rhetoric about how states are on their own, or the federal stockpile is not for you, that kind of quote you see in the news, it's disheartening.

What the future might look like

You could be an optimist and you could start with looking at public health or looking at whether having health insurance come from employers is the right way to do it. But it still kind of goes down to those cultural divides that we've experienced.

Yes, it'll be great to think that we'll have a robust public health system and that the health security system will be rebuilt and that people won't politicize that and the way we talk about it and report it. The media is not to be believed in lots of people's minds, and it's very frustrating to experience that.

The whole thing about public health is that when it's working well, it's not really a story. Nobody writes a news story about a bridge not falling down. That's what public health is about. And it's about protecting the public.

We live in this, "You can't tell me to wear a mask," this fetish of personal liberty makes it really difficult.

That system should be reimagined. Probably health coverage should be reimagined. The federal government's role in all of this should probably be reimagined. So yes, you can be optimistic about it. People might open their eyes, but I think that it's frustrating. Even talking to people in my own family, making that kind of argument and hearing as a response, "Oh, it's not that bad. Oh, people are just trying to make the administration look bad." There's a lot of notions that people have that they're going to be hard to convince, like, "It's not our fault. It's the Chinese's fault."

I'm not sure how that's going to be overcome. I think you do it on a community level. You do it in your own backyard to start with to some degree.

What will happen next?

I think if we're lucky, we'll see a vaccine early next year and if we're even luckier, people will want to get the vaccine, which is certainly not to be assumed.

From my point of view just at work, we're going to see so many changes just because the way we treat patients is different, now. The way we bring patients to the hospital. The use of telemedicine is a whole other conversation which is not going to go away. The way we see patients in the ER. All these things are not going to go back to the way they were.

I think that we're going to be living with it as a chronic illness. And we'll hope that it calms down when there's some sort of vaccine and we can go to work without two masks and an eye shield on, but that's not anytime soon.

Hard Choices

Richard Jenkins

Richard Jenkins (a pseudonym) is a board-certified medical doctor with a specialty in kidney medicine. He was a nephrology fellow (a kidney specialist in training) at a Manhattan hospital when the COVID-19 pandemic struck New York City.[9]

A TYPICAL DAY *in the surge of April 2020*
We'd come in around 6:30, 7:00 a.m. In the ICU, usually I went through my list and look at who died that day. On a typical day, maybe every week you'd lose about two people or three people off your list. Here it was more like two or three people every night. And you kind of had an idea of who you thought was not going to make it.

You start by going through your list and seeing who's missing and say, "oh boy, okay, so those people died." Kind of not really have time to deal with that, because you have to then look at who on the other renal fellows' lists ended up in the ICU, anyone new from overnight, and establish your list of patients for that day. Then you do this whole whirlwind tour of everyone's latest vitals, latest labs. You look at their notes to see what kind of events had been going on over the past twenty-four hours. And the whole time, you have your pager there, and you're getting paged with either new patients, which are going to take a good hour of your time to really research and figure everything out, or the team's kind of panicking about lab values, and they're asking for advice or paging, saying, "Hey, I think we need dialysis, when are they going to get the dialysis?" So that's the morning.

In the beginning we'd see all our patients, that's what we always do. But mid-April, we started not actually seeing people, if we could avoid it. With the whole PPE shortage, what was happening was that if you worked in a unit, you'd have your gown, you'd have your mask, and you kind of kept it on you the whole time, and that was it. That was what you did.

Not everyone on our list had COVID-19. Most of them did, but not everyone. And we also were running around between ten different units, because we're just seeing anyone in the hospital with kidney issues, as opposed to being assigned to one unit.

If we put on an N95 we'd have to get rid of it the moment we saw the patient, because you don't want to be dragging the mask that you wore in one room to another room. I mean, we'd basically be vectors. And we were also scared of getting it, no lie.

So we basically tried to limit how often we would see the patients. We'd rely on the physical exam of the primary team taking care of them, and if we felt that there was something that would change in our management, if we physically saw them, then we'd go see them. If there was something like a real hardcore debate and disagreement about how much extra fluid they had or not, we would see them, because at that point, we need to justify our point of view by actually examining the patient.

Whether we saw everyone or some of them or none of them, I'd then convene with the attending. We'd sit down, go through all the patients, go through the plan for the day, any things we felt needed to be changed with their IV fluids, with their medications, whether they needed dialysis or didn't need dialysis. If they did need it, was there anything special that we had to consider, given everything else going on?

Then the next step would be to call the teams, notify them of what we're thinking, then go to the team, depending on how busy we were, tell them our recommendations. We talked to our dialysis charge nurse, and mentioned who we think needs dialysis that day, who should wait for tomorrow, who needs it immediately, who can wait a few hours. And that's the typical day.

And all through the day, the pager is going off nonstop with more new consults that you have to look at and talk with the attending and see them, and figure out what to do, and constant questions about, "Wait, what should we do here?" Or "Wait, I know we said we weren't going to do dialysis, but look, their potassium level went up, and they're not making any urine today, and I'm getting worried, and what do you think?"

Really extremely busy, not any moment to breathe. I didn't eat anything or drink. It was just work nonstop.

But the worst part of the day, by far, was around 4:00 p.m., where normally our shifts end at 5:00, and we sign out to the nighttime nephrologist who deals with everything overnight. That's a really awful role to be assigned to. Luckily, I never ended up having to do that.

But at 4:00 p.m.—and this is not something that happened before COVID-19—we would end up with a situation where there were ten or fifteen patients that were supposed to get dialysis that day, that we all agreed needed dialysis, that there were not enough nurses to do. As simple as that. Maybe they could do about three of them, but the other twelve can't be done.

And at any moment, you can get a call about another case that might be more emergent than any of those, and then that pushes even those three that were going to get done. And that really, really, really sucked, because that wasn't medicine anymore.

That didn't feel to me like you're being a doctor. It felt like you're doing triage, but when you're triaging between fifteen people that are all cared for by different kidney specialists that are all running around and are not really available, and you know that you're going to be pushing people to the next day, and some of those people—I mean, I can't think of one case that definitely died because they didn't get dialysis the day they were supposed to, but I'm sure that happened.

But that, for me, was the toughest part of the day.

And these decisions, we're using clinical judgment, we're looking at the labs and their oxygen requirements and all sorts of things to decide. But you're dealing with four or five other nephrologists that each are carrying twenty people, and you're all trying to just figure this out. And it was really rough. And there definitely were times when it did become arbitrary.

It just was random. And, you know, I cried a lot when I would walk home after that, because it felt awful. It felt like it's not really what we trained for, it's not what we signed up for.

The intensity of the surge forced improvised solutions.

There wasn't a lot of time then to reflect. Coming up with ideas and solutions—that was where all our minds went. We didn't really want to think about what was happening, just more of what we could do to make it not happen as bad.

This was a problem with patients in every New York City hospital that needed dialysis. But what we ended up doing is, things that we had never done before, really crazy things. Most dialysis sessions are supposed to be three to four hours. We started cutting everyone to two and a half hours, which is not enough—and the thing about dialysis is, the time on dialysis makes a huge difference in terms of the adequacy. It's actually a big deal to lose thirty minutes or lose an hour of time on dialysis.

We ended up with the common good mentality. Not every individual person was getting greatly efficient dialysis, but we were limiting the amount of people who had to get pushed to the next day, so that more people were at least getting something. So that was one big change, we started putting everyone for two and a half hour dialysis sessions.

We change the dialyzer membranes, which we don't usually do because there's always a risk of creating a bit of disequilibrium in the patient, which can mess with their blood pressure or cause certain problems. But the idea was, they need dialysis, but they're not getting it. Now when they do get it, it's going to be shortened, so we need to make it as efficient as possible, even though high efficiency brings some risks. So we started doing that.

Doctors who had previously gathered in meetings communicated by Zoom.

It was really cool, in a weird way. Normally, any change or any big decision just comes from the top down. But because we as fellows were the ones really giving the patient care the most, they would take our ideas and they would actually listen. And they'd let us bounce things around, including all this stuff we're talking about, like limiting the dialysis time, and getting an acute peritoneal dialysis program set up.

Also, there's this giant WhatsApp group, where all of my coresidents that finished our training program for internal medicine were shouting ideas and stuff, and experiences. I actually sent some screen shots to my brother, because I thought he'd be interested. It really got nuts. Everyone was just talking about things.

"What if we tried this?"

"Guys, why don't we try this? Let's do this."

Or, "I heard that they tried this in this hospital, and I actually saw it work here. I think we need to do this, or do that."

A lot of horror stories got shared, too. In one hospital, they had so many people having cardiac arrests from low oxygen that their oxygen system broke down in the hospital. And they had to call an engineer to fix it in an hour, or immediately, and all the people who were on ventilators, because the machines were useless without the oxygen, they had to actually take a bag of oxygen and squeeze it in order to apply oxygen into their mouth. And they called a bunch of medical students and residents to come in and just stand there and squeeze the bags to give them oxygen, which sounds like something in a Third World country. That one stuck with me.

By May 2020, the worst days of the surge were beginning to seem like the past.

It's definitely much better than it was before. We're in this weird limbo right now, because the hospital cancelled all the elective surgeries and all the typical things they do. We've had a really bizarre lack of typical medical emergencies. We're not seeing as many car accidents, we're not seeing as many heart attacks and strokes. I don't know if people are just afraid to come in the hospital, or what it is. But we're slowly starting to see a trickle of the normal stuff we're used to.

But there's still a good amount of COVID-19 in the hospital. We're not getting a bunch of new COVID-19 admissions, but we're struggling with a lot of the people who came in with COVID-19, ended up on a ventilator, .ended up on dialysis, and are now on their horrible fifth week ICU course, unable to come off the ventilator with permanent kidney damage, with neurological damage, when the family still has hope that they'll wake up, and we don't really think so.

We're dealing with a lot of that right now, on top of seeing things slowly come back to normal. So it's kind of a really weird place. It's different than it was in the peak, but it's not normal.

What he sees on social media.

I'm on Facebook. I've got a lot of friends with different back-grounds, and I'm seeing so much BS going around that is so frus-trating to deal with. I follow certain science groups that I find interesting. And they've turned into ridiculous battlegrounds in the comment sections. You have a lot of people that feel that the mortality rate is overestimated, and then when you ask them how they know that, they say, "Well, because they're calling every death COVID-19, even if it's not."

I know everyone who does the death certificates. I work with these ICU physicians. And I have not seen one person ever fraudulently put COVID-19 as a cause of death when it wasn't. And it's frustrating to see a large segment of people really believ-ing this, and believing things like that when I see with my own eyes that that is not true. And that's definitely been very frustrat-ing.

I never imagined there would be a situation where health care workers get lumped into a group of people that are lying. It already happens to some extent, when people are upset about the health care system. But to see it happen with this pandemic as things are evolving, that's something that's really frustrating.

And you can't really convey it to people because they're not there. They're not seeing what we're going through. And I'm okay, like, I'm sad, I've cried a few times.

But there are definitely friends of mine, other people that are not doing so well mentally through this. And I just kind of think of it as spitting on their face, when people say things like, "Oh, they're just lying on the death certificate, it's all just manufacturing this and that." It's not. And it's not even a debate. It's wrong. You can say grass is pink, and that'll be the equivalent.

Everyone just seems to be really fighting and losing their minds. It seems like there's the solid "this is all a hoax" crowd, and I hate them. I hate their guts.

There's the people who are, like, "Well, it may not be a hoax, but it's the same as the flu." And while I don't hate them, they're wrong and I know they're wrong. And you can try all you want, but people are going to feel what they feel, and that's it.

And then, you have the whole attention to the economy. A lot of people are saying, oh, the cure is worse than the disease, and when is the lockdown going to end?

I'm not an epidemiologist, so I don't really know when things should open up and when they shouldn't. But I get it. People are not able to pay rent, people are not able to pay bills. I'm fortunate in that that's not something I'm dealing with. I'm not worried about my job, and I think most health care workers are not *that* worried about their job.

But at the same time, in the middle of a really bad day in the hospital, I'm, like, "I would kill to be stuck at home doing nothing right now."

Coping with Gallows Humor

Steven Palmer

Steven Palmer, a physician assistant at Columbia Medical Center, reflects on the role of gallows humor in helping hospital workers endure the surge in the spring of 2020. In the face of fear, disease and death, he recalls, "it would slice the tension."[10]

EVERYTHING WAS 100 PERCENT COVID-19. For several months.

Our whole unit, me as a physician assistant, and then Rusty Greene, nurse practitioner, and Marvin Castellon and Brit Sovic, research assistants, were all deployed to COVID-19, working on that front completely.

It seemed like this immeasurable nightmare that was going to take us all over.

Rusty Greene, nurse practitioner, was the first person to go to the OR ICU of all of us. He had just gotten back and he was standing at my door and he looked at me and said, "Have you been to the OR ICU?" And I said, "No."

He gave me the fisheye and said, "It's like a horror show. It's a horror movie." I just laughed at that moment.

A once-routine walk from one part of his hospital to another could produce a bizarre juxtaposition that led to laughter.

There was one time that I was going over from the Harkness Pavilion to the Milstein building, to collect labs on a patient who was going to be in our study. As you cross over, the catwalk brings you to the second floor of the Milstein building, and you're able to look over either side to see the lobby of the Milstein building.

On the right hand side you see the gift shop, which was closed down. And behind the gift shop are large plate glass windows that looked out to two refrigerator trucks, where they were storing the bodies of people who had deceased.

As I'm walking by, I'm seeing the refrigerator trucks but then I'm noticing that right in front of the plate glass window in the gift shop I see this large stuffed giraffe. It was this eerie, weird sense of things that perhaps were once meant to help bring you joy or happiness and now meant nothing.

In my head, I knew I was going to be bringing this story back. I was already formulating it into a bit of a comic moment.

When I was talking to another colleague I said, "Gee, I went across and I look to the right and I see the plate glass windows with these refrigerator trucks. And then I looked and I noticed there's a big stuffed giraffe in front of them."

And I knew by my delivery it was funny. She put her hand over her mouth and bent her knees and went all the way down to the floor, laughing. I don't know that the image of a big stuffed giraffe in front of refrigerator trucks translates, but everybody who heard it laughed quite a bit about it.

In a zone of death, an errand to collect blood samples from a patient brought up memories of war movies.

I went with Brit, who was a research assistant at the time. It was always good to bring a colleague with you because they could help you navigate what you needed to do, putting on PPE, bagging the labs, etc.

In front of each one of the rooms were little shelves that had all the face masks and the gowns and gloves, the face shields, and everything that we needed to go in. We stopped in front of the room and, I let out a sigh.

Brit was standing there and I leaned forward, bent over to take my ID chain off from around my neck. As I handed it to him I said, "Here's my dog tags, give them to my kids. "

Brit laughed then and if I bring it up Brit will laugh now. He would bring it up often, hysterical.

The tension of the potential of death or going through some terrible, unusual sickness could affect you. You're just scared to death, gallows humor would slice the tension around it. It seems irreverent. In fact, it is irreverent. We were making light of death. And when you're making light of death, you're inadvertently being irreverent to the people who are dying around you. But it worked. It helped break some of the tension. Almost like by mocking death, we had a power over it, even though we didn't.

Gallows humor is an absolute must. Now when I look back at MASH, I recognize that it was an entire series based on gallows humor. It's funny and it helped.

So much of the time we had to be, forgive the term, dead serious about the work. It was quite regimented. We had to keep moving through in the face of terrible fear, and a lot of death.

You're in the trenches, and you're going forward, and you're on a mission.

Gallows humor was a way of taking that linearity and breaking the hold it had on us. Allowing that heavy duty energy to spill out into a different zone that allows you to relax a bit, allows you to recognize that we're all going through this together.

And one of our ways of surviving with each other or, being colleagues with each other that helped increase that bond, was to laugh.

Palmer reflects on how he uses military metaphors in his COVID-19 stories.

I feel self-conscious about doing that; odd to say since I did it so often. And now in particular because the urgency and the fear of that time has worn off a lot. I feel even more self-conscious about it.

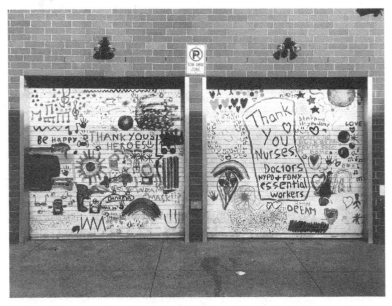

FIGURE 5
June 15, 2020: signs and murals appeared throughout New York City thanking frontline workers, first responders, and health care professionals. Photograph by Naima Rauam, Corona Chronicles Collection, City Lore Archive.

But there was a security person who I met up on the street who said it was like being at war and I just I knew what she meant. And it didn't feel wrong to say that.

I used to use the analogy of being at the storming of the shores of Normandy and you're supposed to run toward the bullets that are coming at you. It's a metaphor. And of course, I wasn't at the shores of Normandy. I do recognize that in total deference to people who were in the military.

It did feel like we were asked to be running into the middle of something that could kill us. Being asked to go forward in the midst of the potential of death just aligns best with military metaphors.

3

Work Turned Upside Down, Spring to Fall 2020

While the nightly cheers of the spring surge focused on health care professionals and first responders, there were other workers whose labor sustained the city that were almost invisible. Transit workers kept buses and subways running so that nurses and doctors could get to work at hospitals. Grocery store clerks and pharmacy staff kept the city supplied with food and medicine. Restaurant workers prepared meals and delivery workers brought them to people's homes. Jobs that once carried relatively little risk—like working behind a cash register—now carried the threat of infection and death.

Even those who could work from the safety of their home saw their work turned upside down. Teachers—who normally rely on direct human connections to engage and instruct students—struggled to put their courses online and to carve out a quiet place to teach from their own homes—sometimes with their own children nearby. They were often working with students who lived in homes where it was hard to find a quiet place to study or join in a discussion amid the cacophony of family life.

Much of the work that sustained the city was performed far from the limelight by immigrants, women, and people of color. The gap between recognition and suffering was particularly acute for transit workers. As early as January 2020, Local 100 of the Transport Workers Union was meeting with leadership of the Metropolitan Transit Authority to discuss how to respond to COVID-19. The MTA had plans in place, but they were inadequate. Workers requests for more protective gear were rejected because the Centers for Disease Control did not, at the time, recommend that healthy people wear masks. Workers who obtained and wore their own masks were told to remove them, the *New York Times* reported. Even when the Transit Authority did double down on worker safety, many of its efforts involved cleaning buses, subways, and stations in the belief—since disproved—that COVID-19 spread on surfaces like subway turnstiles and bus seats.[1]

By the first week of April, forty-one transit workers were dead and thousands were sick. Essential workers still relied on mass transit to navigate the city, but overall ridership plummeted.[2] And the surge in cases of COVID-19 that defined the spring of 2020 was far from over.

Forgotten Frontline Workers

Re'gan Weal

Re'gan Weal is a bus operator and a member of Local 100 of the Transport Workers Union.[3]

DRIVING A BUS *during COVID-19*

There was no traffic. We weren't picking up people. I've never seen Times Square empty. I mean, when I say empty, there were no parked cars at all.

We still had to stay on schedule. A lot of us had to park our buses and wait before we could go to the next time point. We still couldn't be ahead of schedule.

We didn't really have a lot of passengers. But when we did sometimes it was a challenge to get them to keep their mask on. You would have some people coughing and sneezing and that worried us. Most cooperated but some didn't. If someone didn't cooperate, we would call it in, because we didn't feel safe. They would send a supervisor to us or sometimes we could put the bus out of service because it just wasn't safe for anyone if someone refuses to wear a mask.

I had a man who came through the back door, sat in the back, and he was just hacking. He refused to put on a mask. The passengers asked him, I asked him, so I had to call it in; a supervisor came, put them off the bus.

The Port Authority bus terminal was a difficult stop.

We would pick up the homeless when Port Authority kicked the homeless out. They had nowhere to go and at that time it was still a little chilly. So they would come on the bus, which was kind of unsafe for us because now you have the mentally challenged on the bus as well, you have people who you don't know, and you can't predict what they're going to do.

I had one guy who made me nervous because he would just stand there and stare at me in the mirror. And he made me nervous to the point where I called it in. I didn't know what he was capable of. I didn't know what he was going to do. And I wasn't risking it. So I called it in. What you have to remember is that there wasn't really a lot of people on the bus at that time. It was just him and I. And I wasn't taking the chance. So I asked for assistance.

Conditions eased toward the end of the summer of 2020.

At that point everyone was required to wear a mask. Some people were going back to work at the time, but the buses and the streets weren't as crowded as they used to be.

The traffic was great at that time because we had nothing in our way. The streets were mainly empty. So we really didn't have a lot of challenges with traffic. COVID-19 was horrible, but the driving was great.

Honestly, I didn't have to beep my horn at anyone. No one was in my way. I didn't have to worry about anything driving wise.

The mood of transit workers

We had a lot of people die from COVID-19, which was very sad. We were the city agency with the most deaths.

I knew a few people who died and it was shocking. It was disturbing the way it just came in and wiped out over 125 workers throughout the system.

A lot of us were angry. We were frontline workers. We were essential. But people really didn't consider us essential. We didn't matter.

Fire department, nurses, the police department, any city official, they would be mentioned. We were never mentioned. We didn't get to work from home. Nothing changed for us. And we weren't acknowledged in any kind of way. No one cared when it came to us. We didn't receive the respect we deserved.

Bus operators took it upon themselves to stay home because they had families.

A lot of operators slept in separate rooms or they slept in another part of the house.

But other people didn't see their spouses, their children, because they didn't want to infect them. They didn't want to take that chance. So they did what they had to do.

I have one friend of mine who said he had to stay in the basement, basically live down there. His wife would not allow him to come to the rest of the house.

Why people forget transit workers

For the life of me, I don't understand. It is very annoying to us. Because if it wasn't for us the nurses, the doctors, the pharmacists, the essential workers, whoever was needed, they were not getting to work. We were here, we got you back and forth to your destination, safely. And for the life of me, every time there was an interview we didn't receive any acknowledgement from the city, we were never a part of it.

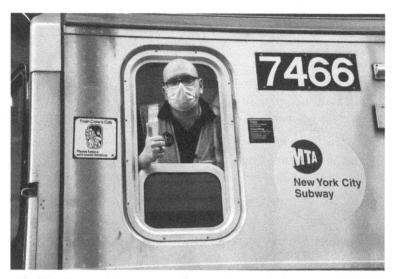

FIGURE 6
August 7, 2020: the Metropolitan Transit Authority begins to install decals on buses and trains directing passengers to remain a safe distance from transit workers. Photograph by Kevin J. Call, MTA.

We Have to Help Each Other

Ralph Rolle

Ralph Rolle is an international drummer, producer, and vocalist. A Black businessman, in 2020 he was the co-owner and proprietor of the Soul Snacks Cookie Company and the Soul Snacks Café in the Bronx. He was on tour with Nile Rodgers and Chic when COVID-19 struck; he immediately returned to New York City.[4]

WHEN WE WERE getting reports during the early days of the coronavirus, some of the information was not given to us for political reasons. One of those political reasons was that Trump was more concerned about himself than the American people, and he didn't want people in the United States to panic by saying the virus was airborne. As the president, you find a way to get the message out without causing panic or hysteria. That's what leaders are supposed to do.

I decided at that moment that this wasn't good. We might want to close our businesses until we get the right information. I didn't want to jeopardize my staff, my family, and myself. So, we shut down and stayed home. I'm glad I did because the COVID-19 numbers started going up pretty fast, especially in the Bronx.

Fauci was giving us his best rendition of the truth. You can see Fauci trying to play political pool because he had a foot on his neck. And I say it that way because I know there were people higher up trying to benefit themselves more than the country, and that's why we are where we are now. To me, it was a great thing to hear Cuomo try to get people on the same accord. He was on TV every day, caring and doing his job.

I started to prepare to keep my family home for an extended period of time. I bought canned foods and supplies so we could be at home for an extended period of time. I got some fun foods because I have a seventeen-year-old daughter, and I didn't want her to get cabin fever. We put a milk crate on the kitchen table and filled it with all of the fun stuff we could think of.

Items in my restaurant that can easily perish had to be given away or thrown in the garbage. We probably threw away about $2,500 worth of product. The things that we could keep we kept frozen. The food items that only stayed fresh for certain periods of time we either ate or gave away.

Rolle shut down the Soul Snacks Café from March to May 2020. He and his wife both contracted COVID-19.

If you care about your neighbors and you care about your family, then you'll make the sacrifices. That's why we closed the restaurant and the cookie company. But what a big sacrifice. I put a friendly note on the front door of the restaurant telling people why we closed. I got some responses saying it was very caring of us to say those things. But that was just how I felt.

I thought COVID-19 was worse than they were saying, and that's why I shut down. The restaurant was just beginning to grow. We were very excited about the numbers that we were getting. And then it all came to a crashing halt.

For me, it was very important to think of safety first. It just didn't feel like keeping the doors open was going to benefit us personally. But closing was very tough. It was tough for my employees; it was hard for us. I kept thinking about them not having any income, so we looked at other stores to see how they were dealing with being opened, like the delis in our neighborhood.

June 2020: The hard work of reopening

The delis started putting up plastic partitions. I thought, "Oh, that's a good idea. We can reopen if we do that." And that's what we did.

I didn't want to put people in jeopardy. You know, this was very concerning to me not to infect people unknowingly.

Americans are not really known for wearing masks. That's something I see when I travel to Japan and all the time. If someone in America has a mask on, people immediately think, and before the pandemic, that there was something wrong with them. And now, if you see someone without a mask, you look at them like they're an alien. Assimilation is an amazing thing.

To reopen, we bought $2,500 worth of food. We had to get everything in place again like we did when we originally opened. We cleaned extensively from front to back. Three days it took us. Each day was about an eight-hour workday of cleaning, sanitizing, and prep for the reopening. We put partitions at the front counter. We bought extra gloves. It was seriously hard to find gloves.

The moral responsibility of masks

We made it mandatory before the city made it mandatory that everyone in the restaurant had to wear masks and gloves, which was difficult because when you're working in a kitchen, and it's hot, it's very difficult to breathe through those masks. I had to remind my staff all the time that you have to keep your mask on your faces. Very quickly, people started to get the point.

So, the process of opening and closing was about the same, but the anxiety of making sure that your staff is safe, you're safe, was tough. And the people that come in to visit, you want to make sure that they're safe as well.

I had one situation where a young man came into the restaurant and didn't have a mask. I said, "Brother, I'm really sorry, but you have to have a mask on."

He said, "I don't have my mask."

I said, "Do me a favor step outside for a second I'll go get you one." I went to the deli a few doors down, bought the young man a mask, and gave it to him. All of the masks in the restaurant, I had custom made for each staff member. I never had an incident when someone said, "I'm not wearing a mask, and I don't care what you say."

There is a moral responsibility that all of us need to take heed that this is not all about our personal rights. We all should be responsible for wearing masks.

Foot traffic in the first two weeks of reopening was extremely, extremely slow. Most of our orders came through our apps—Uber Eats, Grubhub, DoorDash. Slowly but surely, people started coming in. We would get a line out front every now and then. But it was tough going. We needed more people to come in.

What I see is that people are following rules when they come into restaurants, and people are wearing masks outside. But sometimes, when I go past the parkway near Fordham, Mosholu Parkway, there are many people out on the parkways, barbecuing and having parties with no masks. They're not social distancing at all. And I'm always astounded. I'm always amazed to see people out on lawn chairs sitting right next to each other, just chatting away like nothing's wrong. That's scary to me.

But that had a lot to do with the fact that we're not getting solid, cohesive messaging from the top. And just to make a comparison: if this were Obama, it'd be nothing like this. Nothing! He would be responsible for every single person, dead or alive. I think he would've been better for us as a country at that time.

Looking to the future

I'm anticipating a second wave. If we do not get a vaccine, many will die during the second wave. It will probably be worse than the first. At least our first responders will be more prepared, but they will be exhausted. They're exhausted now. And it has all to do with the fact that we need to wear masks. We need to really try our best to cut down as much as possible on spreading this virus to other people.

I do travel a lot. Because I live here, I see this sense of separatism amongst people based on attitudes. When I go to other countries, I see people paying attention to the rules. I think that we have an arrogance that is going to end up killing us all.

I'm a glass-half-full person. I'll do what I have to do. I'll volunteer my services. I don't really get anxiety about myself. When I look at my staff, I get anxious because they need a check. That's disturbing to me. I have one young lady here who's expecting a child. I have people here who were planning on moving and getting their own places. Another young man whose girl is about to have a baby any moment. So, I do feel responsible for them.

But I've got to keep a cool head. I really do. Whether I like it or not, I've got to keep cool. I don't have much of a choice. I can't just lie down and cry about it. I've got to make it happen. So, every morning, me and my wife/partner, we get up and come here.

I've never been a "what if" person. Never. What if can actually back you into a corner and stifle your own forward motion. I'm like, "We got to do this. This has to be done. Now."

When we have good days in the restaurant, I make it known. My entire staff is on a WhatsApp feed. If we have a good sale day, I'll put out a blast of how much we made that day and thank them for their work and their dedication to their positions and let them know that you are recognized for what you're doing, and that my partner and I really appreciate them.

COVID-19, and how we react to health issues, will be the new normal. So, from a natural standpoint we're doing what we're supposed to do. We're adapting.

Despite their efforts, Rolle and his staff could not generate enough business to sustain his restaurant. The Soul Snacks Café closed on December 24, 2021. The Soul Snacks Cookie Company survived. Rolle continues to tour as a drummer and vocalist.

More than a Cashier

Elizabeth Petrillo

When COVID-19 struck New York City, Elizabeth Petrillo was a cashier at the Key Food supermarket on Forest Avenue in West Brighton, Staten Island, and a full-time student at St. John's University. It soon became clear that her job entailed much more than operating a cash register.[5]

I STARTED WORKING at Key Food in January 2020, precisely. It was right when COVID-19 came into the United States but no one really cared about it.

Since the pandemic it has changed. We put markers on the floor to social distance. We put up partitions to protect everyone.

For the most part, people listen, but you do have those people who feel it's all a hoax and they don't want to listen. So you have to get rough and you have to keep your composure. You have your good days and bad days.

At Key Food I am known as a cashier, but the job entails so much more than that. At the end of the day, you have to deal with the customers. You're basically like a therapist when it comes to meeting with the customers. I had people giving me their life stories in the matter of a five-minute transaction when they have a huge order.

Sometimes it's exhausting. You just nod your head and say yes, yes.

It takes a toll. It's all exhausting because people don't realize when you work in a grocery store, especially during the pandemic, it's a hard job. You're basically a therapist, a cleaner, a stock person.

Sometimes you're the bookkeeper with how you have to handle money. Someone is giving you a roll of coins. That's fine. You have to take it out of the rolls and count it to make it's accurate. Exactly.

You also have to make sure your workplace is clean at all times because some people are so ignorant. They won't put anything down unless you wipe your station beforehand. No matter if you wiped it five minutes ago and you haven't had a customer, they want to see you wipe it down.

And some people are so impatient. You could be cleaning, putting stuff back where you got the cleaning supplies, and you could have no one on a register. And there'll be a person there when you come back two minutes later and they're annoyed that you weren't on your register.

I didn't get COVID-19, but I'm a person who always worried. My dad has a heart condition. So I've always worried about his health with the pandemic.

When I got a cold (this was like the beginning of March, right before the shutdown happened) the mask thing was optional. So I came into work, and I was the only one who had a mask on.

You're a grocery store worker, you're in the frontlines—like a police officer or firefighter, like a doctor—and people don't see it that way. So I was the only person wearing a mask for maybe about a week.

I wore gloves for a long period of time. When you're wearing gloves for a long period of time, your hands clam up, they get sweaty. And it's not easy bagging with gloves on. They didn't have the right size gloves for anyone, so it was either too small or too big.

I just started bringing in sanitizer, and you just hoped every day you wouldn't get infected.

It was hard to adjust, but I was also relieved because it wasn't only me who was experiencing this. Even the people who were there longer than me didn't understand what was going on. It was a learning process.

A lot of the people I work with actually have families, or mothers and fathers, and husbands and wives. And it was hard to hear the struggles they're dealing with—their kids not going to school and people are asking for extra hours and not getting it. I was perfect with the hours I have, but there were people who needed the hours to have more money because they were broke and they never got it. And then the people who were favored in my job got the hours.

It's hard to work in a place where we cannot tell people they have to wear their masks because we know some people will take advantage of it. And we're just hoping that no one takes this for granted. I hate the masks, but I wear it for a health precaution.

At Home in the Bronx, At Work in Midtown Manhattan

Patricia Hernandez

Patricia Hernandez, a sales clerk and student from the East Tremont section of the Bronx, juggled classes at John Jay College of Criminal Justice and work at a T-Mobile store in the Kips Bay section of Manhattan.[6]

I HAD TO take the train and pay to get to work every single day.

It's pretty crazy. You feel like you are surrounded by COVID-19. At any moment if you touch a pole, or if you lean on a wall or even sit down on the seats, you don't know who was sitting down in that seat before you, or if they have the virus. You're pretty much in fear the whole time on the train. Many times I would rather stand up on the train ride, which is about forty-five minutes, even though there are seats available. I don't want to sit close to anyone for the fear of getting it even with the protection of the gloves and a mask. You're living in fear.

At work, she coped with the fear of catching COVID-19 from one of her customers.

They've placed mats on the floor signifying six feet of distance between customers. And not allowed more than two customers in the store at once.

Many times we've had to pay out of our pockets to buy gloves. The company hasn't provided us with masks. I've been personally just using my own.

It's been an anxiety working because I am a germaphobe. Every single thing I'm just wiping down.

We have a little table where we have a sanitation section. If they need us to touch their phones they have to take a Lysol wipe and wipe down the phone and then pass it to us.

I've had a customer who really took offense because he didn't feel it was necessary to wipe down his phone and I didn't feel comfortable touching his phone. So he left the store.

I work in a residential area where it's mostly White people. I feel like what they come into the store for is not really essential. It's more like, "I need a screen protector" or "I need a case," "I need to figure out an app in my phone."

You deal with a lot. There's been times where our system will shut down and we can't provide an upgrade for a customer. And he's threatened to call customer service and report all of us. Now I'm explaining to him what's happening: I can't do anything. And he's like, "Yeah, yeah, whatever." Just walked out.

The community that I work in, they're just super entitled. You would expect or hope that they would have more sympathy. And they just don't. It's just more upsetting now.

Virtual classes were a challenge for both Patricia and her professors.

I like to learn hands on, like to see the things that I'm learning in front of me. And having to take every single class online, it's been super tough.

Coming home after working eight-hour shifts to do homework or join a Zoom meeting for my professors is super tough. I'm a full-time employee and a full-time student. So it's been super tough balancing for me.

A lot of professors don't have any background teaching online. I have a professor who's never taught online class before. Pretty much took her a month to get everything aligned.

Next semester is probably going to be online as well. I've really debated if I even want to deal with another semester online. Maybe next semester I'll be better at it, but I just don't know at this time.

The Bronx was hit hard.

This has put our community through the wringer. We're really struggling every single day to provide for our families and provide for ourselves and continue to live in this community. I think it's been tough for people.

My sister was working for a big company, and she was getting compensated, but they didn't know if they were going to open again. So they told her that her best option was to file for unemployment. And then unemployment itself: there's thousands of people waiting to hear back and get paid. She herself has gone a few weeks without receiving any payment and that has a lot of stress on her.

We each provide something here in the household on bills. So she's been in a tough situation where she's scared that she's going to miss her part in paying the bills. And I had to go to work and possibly bring the virus in the house where my mother herself doesn't have the best immune system.

So you have health issues, a pretty high risk to getting the virus because I have to continue to pay my bills, I have to continue to help out in the house. I can't not work. I cannot not have income. I've been working since I was sixteen. That's what I have to do for my family.

I know people who have dipped into their savings because they have to continue to pay their bills. Families are struggling and figuring out if they're going to be able to pay rent next month, and if they're going to get evicted. It's got a lot of us in a tough position.

This virus has really affected poor communities, which are mostly filled with Black and Latino people. Our rates of death are way higher than White people, which is crazy to me. It feels like it was very targeted for us and the government is not doing very much to help us and there should be a lot more done for our communities.

In a crowded working-class neighborhoods like East Tremont, it was difficult to practice social distancing.

In the supermarket or the pharmacy, the lines are insane. They're super long. Thankfully the supermarket by my house has done a great job, and has moved very efficiently. But even the pharmacy, my sister was on the line to get her medication that she needs to have every single day and the wait was almost an hour.

It's been very tough getting used to not being able to get everything you need right then and there. The anxiety of being around people and people not respecting the mask rule. It's also been tough seeing a lot of people outside.

A lot of people in my neighborhood are essential workers. You see a lot of people going to work, getting on the train. The trains are packed all the time. People are walking in the streets, not respecting quarantine. It's been tough.

I want to thank all of the essential workers in my community. It's really eye opening that Black and Brown communities have the highest death rates, but we're also where you see most of the essential workers going to work because they have to provide for their families.

In the neighborhood that I work in, which is predominantly White, you don't see that many people outside because they work for bigger corporations or they make a higher income so they're getting provided full pay at home. And they're staying home.

If it's not necessary for you to go outside, don't do it. Try to keep at home, if one person could go out and do the essential grocery shopping or anything like that.

Keep it at a minimum, keep the rate lower in our communities of people affected by COVID-19.

I know that the weather's getting better and it's May and we want to be outside and we want to try to live normal lives but we should stay home right now. Let this time be a time to spend time with your families. Fix your homes or work on yourself. Let this be a time of relaxation. And let this be a time for us to just continue to fight COVID-19 with quarantine.

I think that it is very important for everyone to understand that there are people struggling and people who try and push through dealing with these hard times. We were very unprepared for what came to us and hopefully it does not happen again. Hopefully we can fight this and get through and stay strong.

Frontline Workers in a Restaurant

Maribel Gonzalez Christianson

Maribel Gonzalez Christianson took over The South of France restaurant at 1800 Westchester Avenue in the Bronx after a career in Spanish and English language radio and television. Since 2004 the restaurant, named by a previous owner who vacationed happily in southern France, has served Puerto Rican and Spanish food.[7]

I AM OWNER and operator of a small business, a restaurant called The South of France on Westchester Avenue in the Bronx. We have been there now almost twenty-four years and I do everything from A to Z. Though I have staff, or I should say had staff, I greet, I host, I cook, I bartend, I clean the bathrooms. I do whatever is necessary. Presently I'm even doing deliveries.

We were known as the Cheers of the Bronx because everyone did know your name. It was a very loving atmosphere. It was a gathering place. My place is not just a restaurant bar, but it was very much a community place, a venue where people had their meetings and planning for charitable events. Everyone had their favorite times to go, whether it was for poetry nights or karaoke or for their favorite dishes. It was a place of community gathering. And that's one of the things that we missed the most, I guess.

It's very hard when you can't continue to operate in the same manner, only doing takeout and curbside pickup and some deliveries. The place is empty. And there's a certain sadness to that, that you can't find the same camaraderie. Though the spirit is there, that dedication is there. We still keep our same philosophies. Our motto is, "We do it all for you." And that's always going to be what we do, and we still bring forth that spirit. We deal with people coming in to pick up food, we answer our calls, or make our deliveries.

We tell people, "Don't forget us, we're still here, we're still doing it all for you authentically fresh, and we're still loving and waiting for everyone to come back."

It's heartbreaking because not only am I and the one or two persons that I'm still able to employ, trying to do the job of many, it's heartbreaking because I don't have the funds and I can't bring back and support the staff that myself and my patrons have counted on. It's debilitating. It's exhausting.

You can't be everywhere in every moment. The lack of sleep, trying to still stay vibrant, and go purchase and cook and pack and deliver and maintain and sanitize the place. Make sure that everyone who comes to pick up food knows that the place is clean and safe. All those things are extremely time consuming. And so days have become even longer because you're covering all bases with no help.

Strength in faith

Thank goodness that I'm a person of faith, and I come back to find strength in my faith. And we now have these delivery services in addition, you know, with DoorDash, Uber Eats, which we didn't have before. But it's still a struggle, because you don't know if you're going to be around the next day, so it's mental anguish. At the same time, it's maintaining positivity, bringing forth the best quality product that you can, and trying to fight the system, waiting for help that you're not getting. So, there's a lot of doubt. It affects you emotionally, mentally, physically. But as an entrepreneur, we face that all the time.

And you have to be positive, you have to know that you can never give up, that it will get better. You have to believe you have to have faith and everything that you've poured into the community, the work that you've done, that you've been recognized for, and that other people will come back, that the business will come back. The Bronx will come back and you stay positive no matter what. Never giving up.

I'll give you a perfect example. When some people that we haven't seen in a while are being very kind and supportive to the restaurant and are coming in to order food, these are patrons that have been with us for years. When they come in I've sometimes gotten emotional and I cry at the sight of them, because I can't hug them. I can't shake the hand. I just have to say, thank you for supporting me. You know, we love you still. And, we're grateful for them. We're grateful for their support and not forgetting us. It's heart wrenching in so many ways because you want to stay strong, but you're human, and you miss people. You miss the camaraderie.

And often when I deliver to people, I see so much sadness, I see devastation, I see food insecurity. I see a hunger, which we're also trying to address as a restaurant. And I am giving pep talks like, "Thank you for supporting and ordering. You know, it's going to get better." I'm giving them encouragement. I'm the mother, I'm their sister, I'm their friend. I'm often the only person that they've seen in a long time because they've been in the house. And there are people who are alone, and they don't have conversation. I'm often giving them encouragement, and telling them that it's okay, that the world is out here. We will overcome this. It's a matter of giving encouragement, all the time, whomever you run into.

Hot meals for health care workers

I've teamed up with another lady named Minerva Aponte who's had a GoFundMe page for hot meals for health care workers. And her mission has been to feed the frontliners, doctors and nurses in various different hospitals throughout the Bronx. And she has hired me, and I've been very lenient in my cost and in my effort to bring forth the best product.

Together we have now fed hundreds and hundreds of meals to various hospitals: St. Barnabas, BronxCare, upcoming now North Central and Montefiore. We're trying to address that, that they feel recognized and appreciated. I'm also giving food to the community. Whoever comes to my restaurant, I cook a surplus, and they will get it and that's at no charge.

I believe that you can't live and work in the community without giving back to the community. We always did that when we were open on the normal hours. For the past sixteen years, we provided a free buffet every Wednesday for three hours where we replenished it constantly. Never missed a Wednesday, thank goodness knock on wood, and we often also did it in the summertime on Sundays. On a regular basis with eighty, ninety, one hundred people every Wednesday.

You have to do with what you can and you have to do more on a lot less. Losing 85 to 90 percent of your regular income is gut wrenching. But nonetheless, you borrow from Peter to pay Paul. I come from the mindset when one eats two can eat, where two can eat five can eat, where five can eat ten can eat.

We are Bronx strong.

That's what Bronx people are known for. We are warriors. We are Bronx strong. And so it takes a lot more time to find specials. When you once could buy everything in one location now you have to go to four locations because they have another item at a lesser cost. Takes a lot more effort, which is where the exhaustion comes in. But you do it because you know that they are feeding people. It's very heartwarming, very satisfying.

I am trying to sleep more. You can't operate under the normal hours, then I have to close earlier, so I am sleeping more. But in all of this devastation, there are also a lot of blessings, because you find that you're more resilient, that you're stronger than you may have thought.

When you need to lug that fifty-pound bag, because you have to make whatever money you can—because maybe some of that can go to feed families that can't afford it—you find the strength, you get the stamina, you find the chutzpah, to lift that bag because there's so many dependent on it. I take a little better care of myself, and I've developed a couple of muscles in the interim.

Frontline workers are not only in hospitals, but they are people like myself and my staff, who are risking themselves to stay open to make a meal, deliver a meal. We are risking our contracting the virus, and we're doing it because we're providing a service because we have compassion, because we have the need. And, you know, we can't take things for granted anymore. We realize that essential workers, people that were blind to us before—grocery stores, truck drivers, delivery people—now we depend on them greatly. People have to have a better awareness that we are more alike than we are different. And gratitude is extremely important. And I think that people have to be more cognizant of knowing that every little bit helps, and we're all in this together.

It varies. People go about their business and they just get their food and to them, it's just another day. Other people are extremely aware and appreciative and are grateful that they did not have to step out of their home. They say thank you, they say stay safe. And they tip better. Tipping is important, people do depend on that.

Working for the Apps

Gustavo Ajche

Gustavo Ajche, a bike courier, is a thirty-nine-year-old K'iche indigenous man from Guatemala who migrated to New York City in 2004. Soon afterward he joined the Workers Justice Project, a Brooklyn community organization and worker center for migrants, and worked in restaurants and construction sites. He became a bike courier in 2018 bringing food orders to customers across the city for the delivery companies DoorDash, Uber Eats, and Relay. His primary form of contact with these companies is through their apps on his cell phone, so he often refers to himself as "working for the apps." When the pandemic struck, he was one of an estimated 65,000 delivery app workers in New York City, a workforce made up mostly of low-wage immigrants from Latin America, South Asia, China, and West Africa.[8]

WE'RE ESSENTIAL WORKERS when it's convenient for the apps, and even for the city at large. We haven't stopped working, not since the lockdowns started last March. We were helping the people who couldn't go out to get their food, or their groceries.

It wasn't easy working through the pandemic, it was dangerous. We were considered essential in the sense of sacrificing our own safety for others, but when it came to paying us well, to saying "thank you," to tipping us, or even just acknowledging us as human beings, not just robots bringing food, that's when suddenly we weren't essential for anyone.

Apps grew a lot during the pandemic because more people were ordering in than ever. They started exploiting us to make deliveries more effective. They made delivery better for customers maybe, but it was at our expense. We kept restaurants afloat when no one could come in, and you heard everyone saying, "Support restaurants, order take out, order delivery." But then, who supports us, the people making that possible? So, our answer was to support each other through Deliveristas Unidos.

Apps have basically rid themselves of any responsibilities to us. We're "independent contractors," not employees. When it comes to our obligations to them as workers, we're expected to act like loyal and happy employees—work long hours, drive longer distances, carry heavier orders, and even grocery packages. But if you act like an independent contractor and reject a few orders because they're too far away or too heavy or are in dangerous neighborhoods where the possibility of getting your bike stolen is higher, then I'll punish you and stop giving you work.

Everything they "ask" of us, they do through threats, sometimes veiled, sometimes not so much, and they go from bad ratings to the possibility of blocking us. It's all about incentives, but the incentives are manipulations, there's no other way of putting it. Don't let the name fool you, we're not independent, but dependent contractors. They remind us that with the hit of a button, we can be erased, and it'll be like we never even worked for them because apps own the technology. They control the whole game for us.

Restaurants didn't allow workers to use their bathrooms or warm up inside on cold days.

We were banned from using restaurant restrooms, let alone take shelter in a restaurant while waiting for an order. That may sound like something that may not be the apps' responsibility, but it is!

There's a type of cold that is just horrible, the kind of cold you need actual breaks from. It doesn't really matter how many layers of clothing you wear; the air gets through you. It's tough, your skin reddens, your lips crack from the friction of riding a bike against the cold, and after a while you just want five minutes inside somewhere warm.

Before the pandemic, there were public spaces where we could just take a break, take shelter. But now, that just doesn't exist for us, the pandemic shut everything down. Most apps don't let you pause for more than twenty or thirty minutes, so something as small as trying to find a restroom to use can cost you a bad rating or even getting fired. It was also just so humiliating not being able to do something as simple as just going to the restroom when you're working.

We were using face masks, and we were only asking for a few minutes inside somewhere warm or cool depending on the weather, and we were just continually told "no, no, no," and in rude ways too. We want to stop being discriminated against, because a lot of the times it feels like it's just racism, the way restaurant managers scream at us, "Don't park near the restaurant, don't touch anything, don't stand here, go there, you're blocking the entrance, don't wait inside, stand farther away." It's just constant screaming. It makes you feel like they want you to keep connecting them to customers, but you should be almost invisible, not take up any space, don't be a person.

The pay was unpredictable, and the apps often stole the tips customers gave the workers.

Apps don't pay per hour; they pay per delivery. I bike around fifty hours a week, and I rarely break over $600. You stay on the streets for hours, just waiting for the apps to need you, and they set all the rules to make more money while you as an individual worker face more challenges, more dangers, and ultimately, make less money for yourself but more for the company. They give you what they want, when they want, and it's never enough. Tips and wages were also stolen from us. So many orders I've delivered, I would look at the restaurant receipt stapled to the food bag that I was bringing to a client, and I'd see a certain tip amount, say $10 or $8. But then, I'd look at the app, and the tip would be different. Sometimes half of what the receipt said, or even less. The app would mark a $5 or even just a $2 tip, and I'm just staring at the restaurant receipt and seeing something completely different. And I wish I could say it doesn't happen often, but it happens all the time, and not just to me, but to so many of my colleagues and friends.

Many workers avoided hospitals because they didn't have health insurance and were afraid of huge bills they couldn't afford.

Back in April, I got sick, and many of my friends and colleagues did too. Many of us didn't even know if it was COVID-19 at first, because testing was very scarce and too expensive. I don't have health insurance. As undocumented people, we're scared of hospitals because hospitals mean huge bills we can't afford, debt we know we simply can't pay back.

So it was mostly my wife taking care of me, a lot of home remedies and teas that to be honest—tasted kind of bad. [*laughs*] The bug was especially bad at night, my wife and I called it the nightly monster. I couldn't breathe. In the end, I just braved it out as best I could at home, but in all honesty, it was scary.

I was scared. You'd watch the news and so many people were getting so sick, dropping dead before they could even get to a doctor, lying on hospital beds with tubes down their throats, their families crying and grieving on TV. It wasn't just coughing and being sick, it was all the weight, the psychological aspect of it, the fear and the emotion that came with knowing I had this virus that was hurting and killing so many people in New York, in the world.

I remember praying and asking God to let me get through it, because I started hearing about so many colleagues and friends that were just getting very sick, some ending up in the emergency room without insurance, some even dying because it turned out that they had high blood pressure or diabetes and didn't even know.

People you just never thought would die, just like that, gone. I absolutely couldn't believe it. They were all young, but you know, most of us just don't have money for checkups. When I think about them, I get very sad, because I know they're like me, the kind of people that could have lived if they had the chance to receive medical care, to be able to afford going to a hospital. I was lucky because I got sick, but I didn't die, even though some nights, it sure felt like I might not make it.

Bicycles were frequently stolen and drivers were injured in crashes with cars and trucks.

You'd think that with emptier streets, we would've been safer, but since our bikes are worth something, around $1,000, $2,500, and sometimes even $3,000 if you count the batteries, we have been targeted more and more. They know we have to go up and down buildings, and we leave our bikes unattended for several minutes. They use bolt cutters, or they rob us at gunpoint or knock us out, and they just take them.

For us, it's just not safe to ride back home at night on the bridges and tunnels that take us from Manhattan, where most of us work, to Brooklyn or Queens or the Bronx. We either travel in groups or we just take our bikes on the subway, or even pay for a garage back in Manhattan sometimes. Besides the bike theft, so many cars and trucks park in bike lanes, causing so many accidents that have killed our friends and colleagues.

Most hit-and-runs that have killed *deliveristas* are just unsolved crimes, and one of our biggest fears as workers is just not coming home after work. So many deaths are the direct responsibility of these apps, because you're suddenly forced to ride your bike at a higher speed to meet their artificially small delivery windows, forced to use tunnels and bridges to complete orders across boroughs, forced to prioritize your ratings over your own basic safety. Lately, so many of us have died, and it's tragic.

I was doing a delivery during a very big storm, and I slid off the road. I tried to keep working after that, but I just couldn't move my leg. I cut my knee pretty deep, and it just kept bleeding. I had no choice but to lay off work for a week. DoorDash asked me if the food was okay [*laughs*]. The pizza was not okay sadly [*laughs*]. Apps "remind" you that you're not an employee, that you're an independent contractor and should be responsible for your own bike, that you should buy your own insurance.

In 2020, app couriers accounted for nearly 50 percent of New York City's cycling fatalities, and at least thirteen delivery workers died on the job in 2021. During the summer of 2020, Ajche and other indigenous Guatemalan and Mexican couriers, with help from the Workers Justice Project, founded Los Deliveristas Unidos, a grassroots collective protesting poor working conditions across delivery companies. On October 15, 2020, they demonstrated for their rights by riding down Broadway from the Upper West Side of Manhattan to City Hall.

It was a great day, because so many of us came together. We were all biking down the street, and you'd just look around and so many *deliveristas* were there, and many were telling their friends to join in. We never really expected to have such a big turnout, it was hundreds of us, almost a thousand *deliveristas* biking together and showing up to protest. It was also somewhat improvised, spontaneous. We got the word out that we were marching a few days before because we'd had it, we were exhausted and frustrated with the whole situation of how apps treat us and how they get away with pretty much anything as employers.

I look back at that protest video, and I just get so overwhelmed and emotional, almost nostalgic. We were able to do it together because the core of the protest was having us speak for ourselves instead of letting apps do all the talking. That protest was the very first time we stood up for ourselves and we fought for ourselves. It was incredible. Drivers talked about how we got our tips stolen, how there was no transparency at all with how much we got paid and how it was calculated, how we were being forced to drive longer distances and carry heavier packages without any additional compensation, but mostly without the choice to say no without slashing our ratings or hurting our future access to work.

There's a lot to fix in this food delivery industry, a lot to shake up so workers like me have a chance to make a decent living without facing so many abuses for a salary that's not even minimum wage. Most people don't know how the apps work, and there's many information gaps regarding their basic functioning, how they make money and how they manage us as workers. Right now, we want more representatives and organizations to know about us.

We need legislators because if you think about us against the apps, it'll never be a fair fight. It's like David and Goliath. We're nothing compared to these billion-dollar companies. We know these apps will fight back, they'll try to intimidate us, get their own council members and state legislators to make sure no regulation comes their way. This fight will absolutely be a long and tough one. We need allies, and I think we need faith in each other so other people believe in us too.

I believe in Deliveristas Unidos. We have a strong sense of community, and we take care of each other. The guys I ride with, we're all from the same village in Guatemala, we all know each other, we know each other's families, they're my family too. I think together we can beat the apps because we're only asking for what's right.

I have two kids back home, a boy and a girl, they're going to college in Guatemala right now. Working here allows me to pay for their education and send money back home to my mom too. In the end, everything I've done with Deliveristas Unidos, everything I'm trying to do, it's also for them, for my kids, because I want them to know that in life, if you don't fight for yourself, no one else will.

After more than a year of driver-led protests, rallies, and meetings with local legislators, the New York City Council passed landmark legislation in September 2021, regulating the delivery app industry by codifying Deliveristas Unidos' demands for better labor standards. The six-bill package included compulsory tip and wage disclosures from apps, a new minimum payment per delivery, free insulated bags for couriers, and the rights to set distance limits and use restaurant bathrooms.[9]

Lessons, Survival, and a Public School Teacher

Damien LaRock

Damien LaRock works as a special education teacher at P.S. 148 in East Elmhurst, Queens.[10]

BY THE FIRST *week in March 2020, school conversations about COVID-19 were increasingly common.*

I started to notice that some parents were keeping their kids home. So our attendance numbers started to drop. And then there were more letters that came out from the Department of Education, talking about disinfection procedures being implemented, and the need for schools to establish a quarantine room.

Friday, March 13, was the last day that teachers and students were all together in the school building. My coteacher and I said, "Okay, all right, kids, it's Friday afternoon, we've got the weekend ahead of us. Things are changing so quickly day to day. Take your math book home, take your writing folder home."

The teachers were not sure that students would return to the school on Monday, and they wanted them to have classwork materials with them just in case.

And then it was on Sunday, March 15, that Mayor de Blasio announced that indeed schools would be closed. So the kids did not return on Monday, March 16. But teachers were asked to come back for three days that week to prepare, to get all of the technology in the building set up for distribution.

Nobody really knew what was going on. We just knew, like, immediately we needed to make this transition to remote learning. There was a lot of panic amongst the school staff about how we were gonna do this.

Monday the 16th we were all working from home, communicating with our families, letting them know that we were transitioning to remote learning. Teachers were calling families, making lists of which kids had computers at home, which kids had laptops, which kids had iPads, which kids had at the very least access to a smartphone.

We teachers came back to the building on Tuesday, March 17. We started to gather together packets of work and all of the books that hadn't been sent home. We bundled everything that we could, by child. We put a pile on each child's desk and had everything ready to go for parents to come pick up later that week.

On Wednesday, March 18, we spent the day in socially distant groups going down to the school auditorium. We got a really quick crash course on Google Classroom and how to start doing remote learning, using Google Classroom.

And then Thursday, March 19, we had the parents come to the school, again in shifts from the morning until the afternoon. Each class had a table on the sidewalk in front of the school. Each teacher stood at a table representing their class. They brought down all of their bundles of work for the kids and the laptops that were going to be assigned to anyone who said that they needed one. And we gave out all of the materials. Some parents came alone. Some parents came with their kids. So in some cases we were able to see our students for one last time and, you know, wish them good luck and at least have a little bit of a sense of closure.

A chaotic beginning

Monday, March 23, is definitely seared in my memory because that was our first day of remote learning and it was a very memorable day.

That first Monday was extremely chaotic. My coteacher and I were able to put some prerecorded messages onto Google Classroom and set up some assignments for the kids. But we still weren't comfortable about how to do live lessons. And we also didn't know how to get the kids to figure out how to log into live lessons, because we had no opportunity to train them on the technology that we were now asking them to use from home. So live lessons were not a thing that first week.

I just remember my coteacher and I were on our cell phones all day long contacting parents and pretty much working as IT specialists. We were doing a lot of work, just talking to parents about how to log into the laptop we had given them.

By Wednesday my coteacher and I had successfully logged in all of our third grade students, which was like such a feeling of accomplishment!

As much as we tried a variety of different methods of reaching out—using the ClassDojo app; calling on the telephone; we got other people in the building, the school aides, to help try to contact them—one particular student was just nowhere to be found. It turns out, through the grapevine, I guess the family moved to Texas.

But the child ended up never successfully logging in. So, I don't know if this child registered for a new school in the community where they moved to in Texas, but it was a sad experience to just lose contact with one of our students and not even get a chance to say goodbye and then be really worried about what access to learning they would have for the rest of the school year.

I'm thankful to say that that was the rare exception for most of our kids. We did see that they were able to successfully log in and participate in remote learning.

Conflicts over computers

Once we started to incorporate live lessons into our teaching, we saw lots of conflicts arise: kids who couldn't use the computer at certain times because their parents were trying to work remotely from home. In some cases families have multiple children, so maybe one kid could get on the laptop, but the other child didn't have a laptop to go on to their class.

We would host live lessons, but we wouldn't necessarily have all of our kids attending. We needed live lessons because we wanted to make sure that we could actually interact with the kids to some degree, but we also needed prerecorded lessons that we made ahead of time, so that if a kid couldn't come to a live lesson, they had access to watch something that was prerecorded. But I am happy to say that I think our school rose to the occasion and was able to relatively successfully implement remote learning.

We were happy that we had a lot of days of 100 percent attendance, but there were also many of those days where the kids were technically there—because they might have commented on something, or maybe turned in an assignment—but they weren't present for our live lessons.

When we did live lessons with the kids, it was clear a lot of kids were in very noisy homes. There was a lot going on in the background. So we just hoped that they were able to attend to the prerecorded lessons that we presented. They may or may not have shown up to our live lessons. We were certainly very happy when they did, because we could then have some kind of an understanding that they were at least getting the content that we were presenting live.

There were some kids who really struggled in the classroom who all of a sudden were doing very well with remote learning. I know of one student in particular whose grandmother just sat with him, and all day long, she was his personal one-on-one, and she made sure he did his assignments and she made sure that he participated when we had our live lessons. And he ended up doing really well, and I think he ended the year pretty successfully.

We had kids who transitioned really well to remote learning. We had other kids who were struggling in the classroom who seemed to be doing better because they got support from their families. And then we had other kids who were doing pretty well in the classroom who seemed to trail off with remote learning. So it was definitely a mixed bag.

Epicenter of the pandemic

I think most of our mental energy was really focused on trying to make sure that kids were getting some semblance of a regular education once we transitioned to online learning. But one of the things that was really quite difficult was realizing that our school was near to what became the epicenter of the pandemic in New York. PS 148 is located in East Elmhurst, Queens. And the epicenter was really centered around the Corona/Elmhurst area, our neighboring neighborhoods. So being so close to that epicenter, we started hearing more and more about families who were specifically affected by the virus.

My good friend and the science teacher in our school, David Shwide, fell ill. He went to get tested at the Jones Beach testing center that was set up there. He found out that he was positive and he shared that information very openly with the staff and with his students. He wanted people to know, like, "Okay, if you had contact with me, you need to know I'm positive."

I also sadly heard from my coteacher Julie Spreckels from our fifth grade class that one of our students had lost his mom. His mom had fallen ill with COVID-19 and, I don't know the details of her experience, but it seemed like pretty rapidly she suffered some difficult effects of the virus and unfortunately passed away. So that was a big shock, and I remember thinking, "Okay, we're putting all of this energy into trying to create these lessons and figure out scheduling, and what is it all for when kids are losing parents?"

As a school, we started to have more and more conversations about social and emotional health of our students and what we could be doing to support our families, who in many cases probably weren't all that worried quite honestly about math lessons and writing lessons. They were worried about the effects of the virus and the ancillary effects of unemployment due to everything shutting down because of the virus.

We heard about more and more people who were testing positive in our school community. Family members, students, fellow teachers. One of our staff members shared with us that she had lost her son. That was a devastating blow because it's one thing to hear that somebody had tested positive, but then it's another thing to hear that someone has lost a family member. So our focus at that point really shifted to making sure that our kids were supported in a variety of ways.

One thing that became clear during this period was that there were kids who either were not coming onto our lessons because they were just dealing with a lot at home, or in some cases their parents were trying to do whatever they could to stay employed or find other employment and were just preoccupied with that and couldn't focus on making sure their kids were logged in to Google Classroom.

Sickness and hunger

And then it also became very clear that in addition to families struggling with employment issues, families were starting to express food security issues. I had kids at certain points who would just announce very innocently in the middle of a lesson or when they initially logged into a lesson, how hungry they were, or that they were sick or that they had family members who were sick.

So as a school community, we started to think about what we can do to support our families above and beyond just creating and posting lessons. Our parent coordinator was really key in terms of sharing information about food resources. We tried to do as much as we could as a staff to share anything that we found out about any resource, anywhere in western Queens that was providing food assistance. We shared that with her so that she could share that with families. ClassDojo became a really important app for us. A lot of teachers had been using that to share announcements prior to remote learning, but it became our main mode of communication with our school community.

We would share lots of posts about any organizations that were giving assistance, whether it be financial or food assistance. And then, thankfully, PS 148, as a school, stayed open to provide meals. So we tried to really spread the word that if families were in need of food, go to the school, they were giving out breakfast and lunch. Our jobs shifted very much from being academically focused to being just as much, if not more, focused around helping our kids with issues around food security and just emotional and social wellness.

And we would post for the parents. And we would always get responses from this particular father, like, "I'm trying, yes, I'm trying to help my son. But can you please let me know if he got on? I'm not sure because I can't check on him because I'm in the other room with COVID-19."

Unfortunately, his son caught it too. And he had great spirits throughout the whole process. You know, certainly his attendance was spotty while he himself was fighting the virus, but he got over it and he came back onto class, and he was happy. And we were all really thankful that he and his father got through it successfully.

I was so impressed and so amazed that despite fighting COVID-19, this particular parent was communicating with us on ClassDojo, checking in to see if his son was getting onto his lessons and doing his work.

Supporting parents

A lot of teachers became really good at supporting parents with setting up their technology, so that became a new role—and then also finder and communicator of community resources. Because it became clear that we had many families who were out of work, and now starting to struggle with food issues. So how could you even think about teaching when you know your students are hungry?

Before the pandemic, we had strong relationships with a core group of families that picked up their kids at the end of the day. That was a feature that went away with the pandemic. We had a small group of parents—maybe around six of them—who were really active in terms of chaperoning field trips. So we got to know them really closely.

And then when remote learning came, all of those live interactions vanished. Our parent communication, in a very natural, organic way, decreased. But the frequency with which we were sharing information, sharing posts, texting, using the message feature on ClassDojo, that increased.

There were several parents who became really, really involved in making sure that their children were focused online and would sit with their children through a lot of our lessons. And so those family members, I think they got a better sense of what we were doing in terms of the content of our lessons.

Students learned to create meeting places online.

Kids became very savvy at hijacking our links. We would post a link for a live lesson, we'd present our lesson and then we'd say goodbye. But then we started to learn that if the teachers didn't either watch all of the children individually leave the meeting, or kick them out by clicking the button that removes the participant from the meeting, any kids left over would stay in that meeting and hang out with each other as long as they could.

It wasn't a bad thing at all, but we started hearing from parents that their kids were having these social groups on our lesson links. And we had to be careful about making sure that they weren't just open, unsupervised links. Once we figured out how to manage that, the kids started group chats on Google Hangouts. And they were free to do that.

It's not all a bad thing because they figured out how to get their social time in there. But I can't imagine that it's as good quality as, you know, hanging out with your friends in person, whether it be in school, or at the park, or in the real world. The virtual world is okay for some things, but it doesn't replace others.

We would hear more and more from parents that they thought their kids were online during a lesson, but what they actually were doing was playing Roblox with each other when they should have been watching our lessons or should have been turning in their work. So we had to compete with online video games quite a bit for our students' attention.

The death of a student's mother

Every day you would hear on the news about the number of new positive cases, but even worse, the number of deaths. And those numbers very quickly became staggering.

Hearing about one of my own students having lost his mother was particularly difficult because it was the first person that I knew directly who had died from COVID-19. It was tough because it was not just a statistic.

His father had requested that he only wanted to communicate with one point person at the school regarding the whole situation, our parent coordinator. That was the hardest part, just knowing he had suffered this trauma, but not really knowing how he was doing through it all.

He did not return to online learning for quite a long time. It was about six weeks before he finally got back. And the day that he came back on, everybody was so happy. And the whole class was cheering, and so happy to see him back. Everybody just started smiling and cheering. That was a really good moment.

After April 2020, there were fewer reports of COVID-19 within the school community of PS 148. But the school year ended in June without students and teachers seeing each other in person.

It definitely didn't have the celebratory feeling that the last day of school would have in person. We tried to have a big, fun, live meeting at the end and say our goodbyes.

By the end of the school year, we had all of our systems set up pretty well and things were running pretty smoothly. A handful of our kids had the opportunity to enroll in virtual summer school. So we knew that we would have some kids who would continue to get some academic support.

Our Google Classrooms didn't shut down. They're still there. We've been posting other little videos here and there throughout the summer. We don't have a whole class showing up, but we've got basically six kids. And so it's good. I think for those kids, this is a silver lining that's come out of it, a continued relationship that we wouldn't have had if we didn't have this virtual platform for it.

In the Cloud: *New York, December 2020*

Rachel Hadas

At Rutgers University–Newark, where Rachel Hadas taught English, classes shifted from in-person to virtual in March 2020. From her refuge at her country house in Vermont, she continued to teach by Zoom. This poem first appeared in The New Yorker.[11]

I made a list I can't find now
(where did all my folders go?)
of words my students didn't know.
Turmeric; poultice; fallacy;
cadence; meringue; Antigone;
Last but not least *Persephone*
are just a few that stick with me,
plucked from the poems that we read
(I tried to stay a week ahead)
between September and December.
Many more I don't remember.
But think of all the words they knew
or thought they knew. I thought so too.
Thinking too hard, though, doesn't do.
Words deeply pondered start to freeze—
as when before our tired eyes
Zoom stalls and stops (and no surprise),
leaving a dark screen, a blank hour
to fill with after and before.
Nonsense syllables devour
denotations. *Happy, sad;*
joyful or *lonely; good* or *bad:*
What does this mean to you? I said.
What does *beautiful* really mean?
I asked them as I tried to lean
into the noncommittal screen,

scanning until my eyes were sore
for the soul in each black square.
Were there really people there?
Did each name hide a secret face
sheltering somewhere in place,
some unimaginable space?
Each word they may have learned from me
in Gen. Ed. "Reading Poetry"
carries its meaning quietly
concealed behind the livid glow
of all we learned we didn't know.
Alone together, here we are,
stranded in our shared nowhere,
marooned in space, while, free from time,
meanings proliferate and chime
as words, unfettered, dance and rhyme.

Inside and Outside

Beth Evans

Beth Evans is an associate professor and librarian at Brooklyn College of the City University of New York. During the spring semester of 2020 she went into quarantine at her home in the Marine Park section of Brooklyn with a small group of family, friends, and students. In the weeks and months that followed she tallied the challenges of working during a pandemic and the relationship between her own intimate circle and the world beyond.[12]

THE CUNY DISTANCE Learning Archive writing prompt encourages students to consider, "Do you have sufficient access to technology, software, devices to complete the rest of your semester?" and faculty to think about "how have you made accommodations for students' different degrees of technological access to avoid exacerbating these inequities? How will this experiment impact the accessibility needs of students with disabilities?"

The prompts suggest that faculty are well situated with appropriate and up-to-date hardware and at the very worst need gentle reminders that their teaching should be mindful of their less well-situated students.

As a reference librarian at CUNY I have been grateful that we already have in place a cooperative chat reference service. Chat reference is staffed round the clock, every day of the week, by librarians from universities and public libraries internationally. During this time of online learning, the chat reference desk became the only reference desk available to our library users.

A corporate buyout meant that in the midst of the pandemic at many CUNY campuses chat reference librarians needed to retrain on a new system. The transition had gone reasonably well, but as with all things technological, there were some challenges. A colleague at another CUNY college got logged off from chat when helping a patron because of the limitations of the librarian's home internet connection. I picked up the student's question when she came back on again, but the student asked if I could reconnect her with the first librarian who had helped her.

As I learned later my librarian colleague at the other CUNY college is still using a DSL connection because she cannot get FIOS in her neighborhood. She eventually figured out that she could switch to cell data and to use her own mobile phone as a hotspot when helping students on chat reference. It was not an economical choice, but it was the only one she felt she could make.

Without too much financial burden, I have upgraded my computer speakers and added an alright-ish twenty dollar webcam to my computer monitor. I can now say with confidence that the image you will see of me in Zoom sessions is distorted by poor camera resolution and not a reflection of my aging face.

But nobody appears to be dressed up for these events. How many of my colleagues have confessed to others present at a meeting their own lack of showering and hair combing before one of too many online meetings?

We all laugh together at the joke circulating about the best time of day to exchange one's daytime pajamas for one's nighttime pajamas and wonder if it is really true that men are seated at their computers not wearing pants. (A professor integrated a pants requirement into his fall syllabus.)

My webcam picks up the wall behind me. You will not see an impressive library of hardcover books, accumulated over decades of an academic life. I am a librarian, after all, and rely on libraries for most of my books. Nor will you see an anonymous white wall with possibly one framed print. My background does not include large windows looking out on trees budding early in back of my Adirondacks weekend home. I have also not chosen to protect my privacy with a simulation of a Caribbean Island. I, instead, have an eight foot by twelve foot map of the world.

The experience of seeing myself against this backdrop for the third or fourth time in one day reminds me that I am working at home, and not in my office at the Brooklyn College Library, where several years ago I dragged a diminutive pink settee into my eight foot by five foot cubicle, along with a Japanese screen, to make the office appear more homey.

As she worked to serve students at Brooklyn College and hold together her extended family, Evans noticed the toll of COVID-19 at CUNY.

Before the spring lockdown had even ended, three faculty and two staff at Brooklyn College died of coronavirus. All were loved by someone or other. I am sure those who loved them were ordinary people for the most part.

I knew the two office staff who died, one briefly because of work I did on a search committee at the college, and the other because our lives intersected at many points.

Jay was a man who delighted in meeting people, remembered everyone he ever met, checked in with everyone regularly and died too young at thirty-one. He overlapped with one of my daughters during their high school years, walked into the Brooklyn College Library as an undergraduate interested in exploring the possibility of a career as a librarian, and showed up frequently in an office in Boylan Hall when I accepted a part-time position across campus as a Dean's Faculty Fellow.

Jay sent me one of his typical, thoughtful and engagingly written periodic emails near the start of the pandemic, about a week after the campus had moved to online instruction and two days after the governor called for a statewide pause in all business operations. By this point in our lives, Jay had gotten comfortable enough to call me by my first name, though I still have a cache of his emails that address me as "Professor Evans." He was concerned that I had "stocked up on the essentials" during these "crazy times," and I wrote back to him that I looked forward to seeing him "on the other end of this."

No, Jay, regrettably I will not see you on the other end of this. Neither is any one of us sure if or when we will come to an "end of this."

Jay seems to have had a very long list of folks with whom he took the time to check in on regularly.

A colleague commented to me that learning more about Jay after his death has left her with the surprised feeling one would have who suddenly discovered her loving husband had dozens of other wives. She was stunned at first, even hurt. "I thought I was his special one," she said.

She quickly came to realize, of course, that someone as thoughtful as Jay could only be the same someone who showed thoughtfulness for everyone he met.

The rising toll of COVID-19 at CUNY through the spring of 2020

The lists of those who have passed away from COVID-19 are growing. The publication website *Inside Higher Education* notes on June 23, 2020, three months and three days from the date Governor Andrew Cuomo declared New York to be on pause, that "CUNY now has the sad distinction of having more coronavirus-related deaths than any other higher education system in the country."

A Horror Story with a Happy Ending

Robert Kelley

As vice president of the Stations Department of Local 100 of the Transport Workers Union, Robert Kelley represents six thousand union members: cleaners, station agents, collection agents who gather fare money, and the workers who handle supplies and parts. He lives in the Bronx.[13]

As a man of color, discrimination is not new to me. I got into union work to protect people who can't protect themselves.

Around March I was doing eighteen-, twenty-hour days, I had a lot of territory to cover.

I was going around checking on my people. And we didn't know what this thing was at the time.

The MTA didn't know what it was, and they certainly wasn't providing us with the proper PPE.

In fact, we were advised not to use masks at some point because if the COVID-19 is on your hands and you touch your face when you pull the mask down, you're more inclined to get it. It was a bunch of hoopla.

I did express to them my displeasure about the way of handling of things. And I also gave my suggestions: please stop misguiding my members and telling them that it's better if they don't wear masks.

I fought with them about my people. We tried to be creative, but it was challenging to say the least.

I remember my breathing changed, so I said to my wife, "I'm gonna go get checked out." And I remember going to a couple of spots that was doing testing and they refused to test me.

The breathing just got so bad that I said, "I'm not leaving. The only way you're gonna get me out of here is if you call the police." And they wind up testing me and I tested positive.

I went home that day, they told me to drink fluids. And that evening, I felt like an elephant was sitting on my chest.

So I call the ambulance. And the ambulance came. They didn't want to come in anyone's house, they just stuck the oxygen thing through the door and put it on my finger. My oxygen level was like around 92, 93.

And they said look, if people go to the hospital they're dying. You're better off staying home.

So I struggled through that night but that next morning, it was just overwhelming. And my wife took me to the emergency room. When they took the X-rays I had COVID-19 pneumonia that would continue to spread. And they admitted me.

His first stop in the hospital was what he remembers as "the nightmare room."

They just put you on a gurney with no blankets, no nothing. And you're basically laying there and everyone has severe COVID-19. And as the people deceased, they would put the covers over them. So you had dead bodies around you. It was a horror story.

And I remember saying, Can I just get some water? Can I just get some water? And periodically, they'd honor that. But that's it. The nurses were scared. They came in, they ran out, they didn't want to be in the mix. Because everyone that was in that room was pretty bad off. It was a nightmare.

Finally, I graduated because they came to say "Mr. Kelley, you made it upstairs." So that's when they put me upstairs into the room.

The doctors were coming in and I was asking them questions and they were brutally honest: "People in your condition typically are not making it through."

I refused to take the ventilator. But I was on oxygen the whole time. And being relentless as I am I just fought.

I was sweating profusely. At some point I told them just leave my bedding. I was changing my linens three times at night because I was waking up soaking. But that kept me alive, I truly believe me doing that kept me moving and whatnot. I think that helped my cause.

I remember the struggles. Clearly it was a lot of struggling.

I lost a couple of loved ones who was very strong at the end. And ironically, the crazy part about it was I was good. I looked at the way that I've lived, I looked at my business affairs, I thought of my loved ones and good deeds that I've done in my life, I honestly felt okay. I said, Well, hell, if there's a heaven I got a good shot at this stage.

I spoke to some loved ones once again and expressed to them what I wanted and stuff like that. And it was a very challenging time.

Just before he was admitted to the hospital, Kelley was part of a Cornell University class in labor law; one of his classmates was the president of a nurses' union. As word of his hospitalization spread, nurses took a special interest in him.

Next thing I know, I had everybody coming from all over the hospital. I got so much special care. It was phenomenal. Prior to that all I had was three doctors coming in with masks on looking at me and shaking their heads. They gave me a different breathing apparatus and all that stuff. And we worked through it.

On the grace of God, I'm here today to be able to perform my duties and to be with my family. So it's a horror story that turned into a pretty happy ending.

Kelley's cell phones kept him in contact with his union.

I continued to service the membership. And my partner at the time, Vice President Linwood Wichard, got wind of that. At the end of the day, he took my phone he said no, you're not working. But then I had my personal phone, so I was still working. It was probably kept me going, moving instead of laying there dying.

The cell phone also brought news of deaths.

I had close people that worked with me side by side who died. In fact, our first loss was in management. I've had managers and supervisors that passed away that I knew that were really decent people. And it was very disheartening.

I lost some good friends. I lost a plumber, a really dear friend of mine, sweetheart of a guy. I lost Caridad Santiago, she was a sweetheart of a cleaner. We lost several station agents.

Kelley was released, ran himself ragged working and went back to the hospital and was released again. Altogether, he was hospitalized for a week.

I got to the point where I was able to go home because they had given the room to people that was worse off than I was at the time. And I was willing to go home at that time, I felt confident enough that I would be able to do what I needed to do to keep progressing.

When I came out, the first thing I did was set up a team meeting on a Sunday. Everybody's Kumbayaing and I said, "Okay, here's the deal. Tomorrow, everybody's back to work.

"Let's be careful, let's put our mask on, let's put on a proper PPE, your rubber gloves, whatever you need to make you comfortable, social distance and things of that nature. But we owe it to the membership to provide the protections for them. That's what we all signed up for."

I was always a hands-on guy. The fact that I did see what was probably the other side and the possibilities that I might not be here, I took it as a blessing from God that God says, "You're here for a reason." And he's using me as the vessel for me to be able to continue to be able to protect others.

At the end of the day, I can stand here strong and say that through this pandemic, if I've gotten anything from it, I believe that it made me a better man today.

New Yorkers need to understand the value and moral fiber of what New York is built on. We're a twenty-four-hour bright light city. We're not made for fancy trains and fancy train stations; we have built on New York City strong.

I think that New Yorkers are resilient. I think that we have a way of bouncing back. I think that New Yorkers know that we overcome adversity every day.

I think that the big message was life is short and let's cherish each and every moment that we have on this earth because you'll never know. You'll never know.

4

Losses, Spring 2020

In the spring of 2020, when New Yorkers went into isolation to slow the lethal spread of COVID-19, they were severed from what they loved—and what they loathed—in their city. If it was good to hear the sounds of birds instead of the noise of traffic, it was painful to hear the wail of sirens and count the rising number of deaths. When New York went on pause on March 22, some eighteen people were dying daily. The number grew dramatically until the first week of April, when about eight hundred were dying daily. Deaths then declined sharply until late June, when they were back at the level of late March.[1]

The isolation frayed people's everyday sense of connection, both to their environment and one another. The basic building blocks of social life—seeing people at work, meeting them for drinks or coffee, exchanging a quip on a street corner—all became things of the past, "the before times."

The geography of the city was transformed, too. Even in the middle of the week normally bustling neighborhoods such as Times Square and Wall Street were as quiet as a Sunday morning. Familiar businesses closed when it became clear that they could not outlast the pandemic; heartfelt notes to patrons, taped into windows and doorways, served as epitaphs for beloved bars and restaurants. Playgrounds were closed—until health authorities figured out that the virus was airborne and did not spread by people touching playground swings.

People lost opportunities to gather in groups and celebrate events great and small. Religious worship went online, weddings and birthday parties were canceled. Burials and funerals were limited to a tiny number of people. The cancellation of a long-anticipated event, like a retirement party, suddenly put a blank spot over a date that had been intended to punctuate weeks and years of happy anticipation.[2]

Over time, the accumulated disappointments took a toll. Some people became sad or bitter, others withdrew into a zone of safety. Still others ignored social distancing requirements altogether.

The accumulated weight of these responses degraded what one observer called "our social metabolism."[3] The losses varied with the individual, but over time the monotony of the lockdown could confound people's sense of time, while isolation eroded their capacity for interacting with others and made them less tolerant of human foibles.

Worst, of course, were the deaths. In normal times doctors and nurses could at least comfort the dying, even if they could not cure them. Family members could hold their hands, pray for them, or serenade them as they passed from this life. During COVID-19, however, under a state order, hospitals banned visitors to prevent the spread of the virus.[4]

Nurses heroically tended to patients in extreme distress, but it was impossible to maintain the kind of bedside family visits that eased a person's passing in normal times. The ordeals were summed up in a phrase that gained resonance during the most trying days of the pandemic in New York City: "You die alone."[5]

Survivors lost not just loved ones, but opportunities to grieve and heal. During the worst days of the pandemic, the number of people dying was so great that funeral homes and cemeteries were overwhelmed.[6]

The fear of contracting the virus from a body, and the restrictions on social distancing that kept the number of people at a funeral to a minimum, allowing mourners to watch burials only from a distance, meant that the normal processes of grief were suspended.[7] Stephanie McCrummen, a reporter for the *Washington Post*, recounted how beleaguered workers at the Neufeld Funeral Home in Elmhurst, Queens, stopped organizing traditional funerals and transported bodies directly from the hospital to a crematorium. She called it "death without ritual."[8]

Alfreda Small

Alfreda Small, a member of District Council 37 who lives in Staten Island, worked as a home health aide and as a police administrator before retiring.[9]

Changes to 4 train
Took forever to get home
Tired as hell now

Thomas Barzey

Thomas Barzey lives in the Bronx, where he was born and raised. Currently an actor, he has worked as a stage manager, home health aide, and office assistant.[10]

Afraid to go out
Cannot let anyone know me
Please hide me

Quarantined and Unemployed in the Bronx

Nichole Matos

When COVID-19 hit New York City, Nichole Matos of the Morrisania section of the Bronx was working at a gym and studying at John Jay College of Criminal Justice. She was laid off and went into quarantine.[11]

I WAS WORKING at 24 Hour Fitness, which is a gym in the Riverdale area of the Bronx. I was a service expert. I've been working there for about twoish years.

Once everything started happening with the virus, they immediately closed down; gyms were one of the first places to close. My manager informed me, and they didn't really have much information at first, but then they told us that they would pay us the next pay date, which they did. And they advised everyone to apply for unemployment, which I also did. And they haven't really said much as far as reopening.

I'm genuinely concerned. I'm not sure if I'm still going to have a job. One of my co-workers forwarded me an article about the company regarding their financial issues and possibly bankruptcy, which is a little concerning for me and other co-workers. Are we going to have a job? They're not really vocalizing these issues, which is probably none of our business in their eyes.

Unemployment for me personally has been a smooth process. I was able to apply online and I was able to receive money, which is good. So I can't really complain. But it's just a matter of, "What's going to happen when this is over?"

Nichole quarantined with her mother and sister in Morrisania.

From a human perspective, it sucks. You miss your friends, you miss your family, you miss just having the freedom to do what you would normally. It's now more of a routine. Same thing every day.

You get tired of eating the same thing, watching the same things, reading the same things for class and meeting for these virtual classes. I feel like sometimes it could be redundant and repetitive and awkward and pointless and a waste of time. I could be using those two hours for that lecture to work on a paper or something. I feel that professors—they're trying, but I just would like to be a little bit more realistic. Certain things are just not working.

In the event that we do have to continue to distance learning, I feel like they should work on just how they actually have the classes. I don't think the virtual meeting twice a week, three times a week is necessary.

There are days that I cannot wait for the semester to be over.

I miss having a normal life. I miss going out and just doing stuff.

I know that the program that I usually do for internships is not happening this summer. That affects me and a whole bunch of New York kids. We depend on employment programs and internship programs to keep us doing something educational or just overall positive. If the quarantine is not over by the summer, there's going to be a whole bunch of kids in the streets. There's no benefit of having the freedom if we're not going to be able to have these programs keeping us busy in the summer.

I don't really socialize much within my neighborhood. I have a couple of friends in the building. And they've pretty much been on the same type of time that we have at this household. I know just from seeing outside the window that the streets are empty. The homeless people are definitely out there which is sad and concerning.

Businesses have closed. There was a supermarket down the block, the owner and his wife contracted the virus and he passed away. And that's kind of concerning, because anytime you step foot outside, it's a risk. Even going to get your groceries you have to be extra careful.

In moments like this, you have to make sure to take care of yourself and take these things seriously. The reality is that you can get it anywhere. Doesn't matter the age, doesn't matter the health conditions. It's something that we can't avoid. We have to try our best to be not only considerate of ourselves and our family, but others. There's nothing more important than your health and safety.

Socializing is important. It's needed. It's wanted very much. But you just have to adjust and know that we're going to eventually be free. We're going to eventually have the freedom that we want, but for right now, we just have to focus on keeping those numbers down, as Cuomo says.

Saying Farewell

David Hunt, Tess McDade, and Peter Walsh

In March 2020, bars and restaurants in New York City closed temporarily (except for takeout and delivery) to limit the spread of COVID-19. Over time beloved businesses closed, including Coogan's Bar and Restaurant at 4015 Broadway in the Washington Heights section of Manhattan. Opened in 1985, Coogan's had become uptown's unofficial town hall—loved by residents, politicians, off-duty police officers, and doctors and staff from the nearby New York-Presbyterian/Columbia University Irving Medical Center. In 2018, Coogan's had fought off a massive rent increase with the support of friends and elected officials, but it could not overcome the challenges of COVID-19. In April 2020 owners David Hunt, Tess McDade, and Peter Walsh announced that Coogan's was going out of business. Coogan's became the subject of the documentary film Coogan's Way, *directed by Glenn Osten Anderson, released in 2021, and the book* Last Call at Coogan's: The Life and Death of a Neighborhood Bar *by Jon Michaud, published in 2023.*[12]

APRIL 21, 2020

To our Coogan's family and friends,

We need your help in saying farewell in a message that is so very difficult to write. What's missing are your stories and wishes and even pics that will make whole the heart of our saying goodbye.

Ironically, this past March 17 would be the last time Coogan's closed its doors. We had hoped to open them again but sadly that is not possible.

To all our Coogan's family that extends from a corner in New York's Washington Heights to so many near and distant places, we offer love and best wishes that you remain safe, strong and healthy for now and ever.

Our first priority will be the security and future of our staff. We encourage our friends to contact us to help this quality group of the best possible people in talent, hard work, and integrity to obtain jobs and employment. For over thirty-five years we have given and received more than is usual in a working experience.

What was made at Coogan's were warm friendships, easy smiles and hearty laughter. If you came in a stranger, you immediately became a friend and left as an "old timer." We were able to share a full glass of love with a large plate of honesty in a neighborhood full of the most wonderful people you could ever hope to meet.

At this time we are so proud of our friends and professionals at NewYork-Presbyterian Hospital and Columbia Medical Center who made Coogan's their home away from home. Thank you for who you are and what you do. The world depends on you!

To many of us, Coogan's was a public house, a meeting place, a table to break bread and solve problems. We were a place of celebration and remembrance. We were a bar full of life . . . a place to listen and a place to talk. We were a place to leave behind the burdens of everyday life and, more often than not, inherit new ones when we volunteered to help a neighbor in need, a kid in search of himself, or a stranger down on his luck.

We were people of different races, creeds and ideas, all with the same dream to be secure and love. We were a place to find out you weren't alone but if you wanted to be, your space was sacred. And together at Coogan's we became stronger and powerful, with an urge to share and offer ourselves with deeds that gave us, in return, the realization of life and the essence of beauty.

There are so many people we would want to mention for their consideration and friendship, especially during the past few months, but we hesitate for fear of omitting anyone. That will come later when our emotions are settled.

Now it is your turn to complete our story . . .
Sad and grateful,
Gracias, slainte and thank you
Dave, Tess and Peter

Living in a Shelter in the First Year of the Pandemic

Rozelyn Murray

COVID-19 took away something that Rozelyn Murray treasured: her days at school that gave her a break from living in a shelter. Her essay first appeared in COVID Class 2021, a platform for students in David Rohlfing's English 12 class at Pace High School, a public school bordering Chinatown and the Lower East Side.[13]

MY EXPERIENCE DURING the pandemic was a little different from others' because of my living situation. My mother and I had moved into a shelter in August 2019 after she lost her job. I was very grateful that we had somewhere to stay, but I hated being there. School was my only escape.

Every morning I would wake up excited to leave the shelter and see my friends and all my teachers. After school I would not go straight home, I would stay in the park with friends talking about everything in the world. Going back to the shelter was the worst part of my day, it was such a drag to get there. I would rarely miss school and if I did it was because I had a doctor's appointment.

Who knew that on one random Friday in March 2020, it would be my last day of school? It was very sad to hear the mayor say that we couldn't go back to school because of how rapidly the virus was spreading.

I became very depressed and hoped we could go back to school. I knew that my health and everyone's health in the school were important but I was very adamant about going back to school. My mother and I would watch the news every morning to see if anything changed, but there was no luck.

I knew it was getting serious when the school was sending in work from Google Classroom. At the time I did not have a laptop, so our assistant principal Mr. Chong was very generous and brought a laptop to the shelter. During this time the school was very helpful and so were all my teachers.

The room I was staying in with my mom was starting to get smaller as the days passed. It had two twin size beds, a TV, a bathroom, and a mini fridge. Thank god we were not dirty, we made the room as neat as possible. Again, I was very grateful we had somewhere to stay, but my mother and I started to clash because of how small the space felt.

The only income we had was my father's contributions and food stamps. We could only buy limited amounts of food because we had no space and the fridge was small. There was no stove so all I was eating was microwaved food and outside fast food. I gained a bunch of unwanted weight and slowly started to hate my body.

My life started to feel very boring because of all the eating, sleeping, and watching TV. There was a point where I felt stuck and I felt that we were never going to get out of the shelter. I wanted my own room, a kitchen, a dining room table and just the feeling of being stable.

COVID slowed the process of my mother and me getting an apartment. We waited for a whole year until they gave us keys to our new apartment. That was the most exciting day ever. I was already thinking about life after COVID and having my friends and family come over.

Phone calls with my friends were the best because of all the laughs and all the "remember when" conversations. My friends and I would even talk about how we were going to hang out when all of this would be over. By the time we were able to hang out, our friendships broke apart.

It was very sad to see that over the months of the pandemic, we were starting to grow apart. I would think to myself about how if we were at school our friendships would still be strong. There were many times I tried to rekindle my friendships but it didn't work out. It came to a point when I started focusing on myself and hanging out with friends who actually wanted to be my friend.

I can really say that COVID messed up my whole twelfth-grade experience. It stole the joy from seeing my teachers face to face, hanging out in the gym with my friends, and meeting new people. Going to the prom was one of my biggest dreams and COVID killed it. It makes me angry because why didn't the government have this under control? High school is pretty much over and I waited for this for the longest.

I am very proud to say that even though COVID came around, I was still focused in school and never slacked off. I am very grateful that all my teachers and my mother were huge supporters for me during this tough time.

Grief Works from Home at All Hours

Michèle Voltaire Marcelin

New York is a city of immigrants, and many are haunted by memories of tragedies in other times and places. In Brooklyn, Michèle Voltaire Marcelin—Haitian-born poet, visual artist, and performer—was haunted by the mass graves of Chileans executed during the 1973 coup and Haitians killed in the 2010 earthquake. But nothing prepared her for images of mass graves in New York City in April 2020.[14]

Sleepwalkers confined in a dream
Six feet apart like barbed wire
The days pass by without measure
Calendars have been quarantined

State your name and take a number
Stand in line for time regained
Only the mirror knows your face
The mask you wear beneath your mask

Don't inhale the poisoned air
Pass each other in silence
The ground itself is a peril
Keep your shadow at a distance

Your chest filled with glass splinters
Beware, Beware the crown of thorns
It lights a fire between your eyes
Delirium in Technicolor

Don't break silence with trifling words
Thousands die behind closed doors
Disposed of in mobile morgues
In standard issue body bags

They dig mass graves on Hart Island
Pine trees on which we carved our hearts
In parks where children ran and played
Are now boxes that hold our dead

Sorrow is never on holiday
Misery is not on leave of absence
We've exhausted all appeals
Grief works from home at all hours

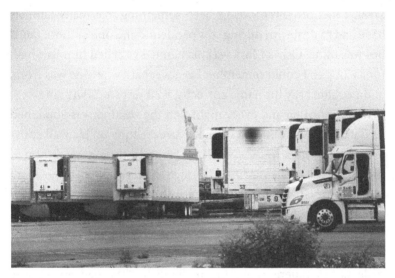

FIGURE 7
May 6, 2020, Brooklyn. Photographer Bryan R. Smith writes: "The Statue of Liberty is visible beyond the refrigerated morgue trailers at the South Brooklyn Marine Terminal. The trailers held the bodies of people who had died of COVID-19. The emergency morgue was set up in April until funeral homes or crematories could accept the bodies. . . . The Statue of Liberty is a symbol of America and to see trailers of bodies at the base is an image of a country failing at the most basic responsibility: to keep our citizens safe. Knowing now what we didn't know then, this photo speaks to the failure of the Trump administration to have a cohesive national plan to address the virus. At the time, I hoped that this image would be a notice to Americans to take this virus seriously, to follow facts and science, and to wear a mask out of respect for first responders and fellow Americans who are putting themselves in harm's way for us."

The Second Father: A Tribute

C. A. Duran

"A Second Father: A Tribute" first appeared in COVID Class 2021, *a platform for students in David Rohlfing's English 12 class at Pace High School, a public school bordering Chinatown and the Lower East Side.*[15]

DEATH HAS UNFORTUNATELY been something that many families have had to deal with during this pandemic and one of those families was mine. Osiris Mora was his name. I've called him San Juan for as long as I could remember because that's where he was from, and I couldn't say his name correctly, so it just stuck with me.

Every morning and every night that the weather was good, he'd be outside his building on Orchard Street sitting on his walker listening to Spanish music on a JBL Clip 3. I'd usually catch him at night because in the morning I'd leave too early.

Osiris was always filled with energy despite having many health problems such as undergoing open heart surgery, diabetes, high blood pressure, and probably many other problems that I didn't even know about. There is a saying in Spanish that goes, "Hierba mala nunca muere," meaning in English, "The bad guys never die." He and my dad were the bad guys according to my mom and his wife.

My dad always called him El Malo, meaning The Bad Guy. For what reason, I don't know, but he wasn't supposed to pass, at least not yet.

There is this one memory I have as if it were today. It was when I was around thirteen or fourteen playing in a little league baseball team called the Sharks. It was a small league in the Lower East

Side neighborhood that I'm pretty sure is still up and running. It's called OLS (Our Lady of Sorrows), and, yes, it's a church thing.

We were playing in Field 4 on a partly cloudy type of day. The field was nice because it seemed like the day before they had raked it and put new sand over it. My parents weren't able to make it since they were off on a little romantic getaway, so I was staying with San Juan and his wife. He had brought me to the field a little earlier so I could get some throwing in with him.

At this time he was healthy for the most part, but was on the verge of running into health issues. I was all warmed up and the game had started. I was a pitcher at the time and that had to be one of the best games I've played. We were tied at the eighth inning and I was about to go up to bat.

While I was warming up, San Juan approached me with some advice. "Keep your eyes on the ball, even when he's winding up. And when he's getting ready to throw, pick up your front leg and swing with what you got." And I replied, "Oh, I will."

I was up to bat and at the first pitch I did as he said. DINK . . . was the sound my bat made when I hit a bomb to left field. I ran and ran. Home run!

I got to the plate and after celebrating with my team, and saw San Juan through the fence with only excitement. I went and hugged him like he was my own father. At least it felt that way. After we were done with the game we got ice cream and made our way home.

While I was on my way back from practice on May 10, 2021, I saw the ambulance at the building door taking down what seemed to be a body in a white bag. The body slid down on a flat stretcher.

I made my way upstairs with confusion and then, as I opened my door, I saw my father with a face of sadness. He told me. My heart felt like it was going to drop out of my body and the anger filled up inside me. My dad's not one to express his emotions, but we hugged each other as we both let tears go down our faces.

I couldn't believe it because the day before, San Juan was sitting listening to his music and I was speaking to him. He was telling me about how life was so short and to make sure I have fun as a young teen.

It's always when you least expect things to happen that they happen. My "second father" gone and we are here having to continue life like everything is supposed to be okay. If I had a chance to see him again I would hug him and tell him how much I loved him and appreciate how much he did for me. May he rest in peace.

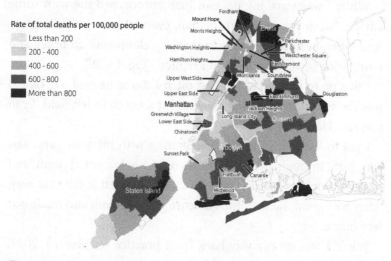

FIGURE 8
New York City death rates by zip code, January 2020 to May 2023. Chart: BetaNYC. Data: New York City Department of Health and Mental Hygiene.

He Was the Block's Papa

Veronica E. Fletcher

Joseph Trevor Fletcher, known to his family and close friends as Trevor, worked at the Flatbush, Brooklyn, bus depot as a bus maintainer group A, responsible for all installations, maintenance, repairs, and inspections of the body, mechanical, structural, and electrical equipment on buses and other automotive vehicles for the MTA. Trevor and his wife Veronica had three children, Joshua, Zachary, and Madison. Veronica, a former high school teacher born and raised in Queens, recounted his life, his death from COVID-19, and his funeral.[16]

IN ADDITION TO being our children's father, he was like the block's Papa. Trevor would watch everybody's kids like he was their father. He would be out there fixing everyone's bikes and watching all of the children that came out to play.

My husband was the kind of man that would save a child's life anonymously and want nothing—no recognition, no credit—and then just go back to whatever he was doing. And not tell anyone. Not even me.

On July 4, 2020, a neighbor stopped me and introduced himself to me and then expressed his condolences while telling me about his family's gratitude for my husband because Trevor saved the lives of both his son and his nephew when the toddlers ran out into the street. Whenever they tried to thank him, Trevor would just buy everyone ice cream.

An immigrant to the USA with a passion for travel

One of the things that was most important to my late husband was travel. He was an immigrant to America from the country of

Grenada. And he wanted our children to be global citizens. So at the age of two months, once they got their shots and passports, each of our three children was on a plane out of the country for their first trip. This was important because my husband said they had to have their sea bath in the Caribbean, just like he did. That's why travel was essential for us as a family.

He wanted our children to know that the world is bigger than Brooklyn, New York, and the world is bigger than the United States. So, we traveled to different continents. We regularly traveled to different countries in the Caribbean and other places. We took frequent road trips, and we took lots of cruises.

One of my husband's favorite trips was in 2009, when we flew to London then took the train to Paris for a few days. He was so excited and proud to show our boys the Grenadian flag in the Eiffel Tower viewing deck.

A job that was a calling

My late husband was an incredibly strong man and he was dedicated to his duty.

Transit wasn't a job for him. It was his duty. It was his calling. Those were his brothers and sisters. Once we began having children every year we would go to MTA Family Day. One time they had it at Six Flags in the rain. I even have a picture of our oldest son in a full fireman's raincoat and our youngest son in the stroller with the rain cover. What are we doing in an amusement park in the rain in torrential rain? Our family was there for a family day. That's who he was.

Early in the pandemic, confusion about COVID-19 and its treatment

For many people it's hard to fathom what it was like at the very beginning. The country didn't really know anything. In New York we were the epicenter. We would see videos of people being hosed down in China, but my husband knew what the general public knew, which was very little.

So, for my late husband, going into work, it didn't matter how he felt. He was going into work. He went to work and did what he needed to do, because he needed to be there in the trenches with his co-laborers, and to make sure the city kept moving. He wouldn't have told me that he did not feel right. He would've left the house saying, "Time to make the donuts. Honey, I love you. I'll see you later."

My children were home doing remote school and my late husband was going to work.

My husband and I took care of each other. My job was to make sure that my husband and my children had what we needed. Everybody had to take probiotics in the morning. I'm buying the easy peel tangerines, and everybody had to eat them. Our discussions were about family and probiotics and vitamin C and washing our hands.

Trevor got sick in March. We never had a discussion of what was or wasn't being done outside of our home. My priorities were how he felt and how I could help him feel better. Any discussions with my late husband were about, "Here's some elderberry. I've got Gatorade. I've got electrolytes. Here, drink more electrolytes. Here's some tea and take some probiotics. Have extra fluids."

When he felt physically ill and could not continue going to work, that's when he sought medical assistance.

And then eventually, the treatments were no longer working. Everything just happened rapidly after that.

The last time that I got to have a conversation with my late husband was March 31. That evening I gave him his medicine and of course some electrolytes and some elderberry and tucked him in.

And he told me he loved me. I told him I loved him. And I gave him a kiss on his forehead like he always gave me. That evening at about seven was the last time I heard my husband tell me he loved me.

Early the next morning I found him in respiratory distress. Choking. Having difficulty breathing. And that's when I called the ambulance, April 1 at about four in the morning.

That's the last time I held my husband in my arms. And even in that moment I did my job, cleaning him up because the mucus was coming out. I cleaned him up and I talked to him and encouraged him, told him how much we loved him and needed him.

It was trauma for our entire family. Our children, all of them, saw the strongest man, their hero, the strongest man in the history of men, in respiratory distress, fighting to breathe and fighting to hold on to his life. And he did that for us. Like a valiant warrior and soldier. For eleven days in the hospital he fought for his life and fought to come back to us.

He was intubated. I had opportunities to interact with my late husband through FaceTime videos.

More than once, doctors would call and say, "Hi, Mrs. Fletcher, I'm going to call you back so you can say goodbye." I received several of those phone calls before I received the last phone call.

The last words that anyone said to him in our family were on April 11 when I gave my children an opportunity to have their FaceTime visit with him. They told him that they loved him and they needed him. I chose to let those be the last voices that my late husband heard of anyone that he knew. I'm sure he heard what was going on in the hospital with the doctors around him, nurses and what have you. But he also heard the love of his family. Instead of it being me talking, I chose for it to be our children, so that way they could have their last moments with their Papa. Knowing and loving this man almost twenty years, they wouldn't get that twenty-year opportunity and I wanted them to have that memory and that knowledge that their voices are the last voices that their Papa heard of anyone that he knew.

At that time at funerals you were able to have ten people in person. The casket was closed. I was never even able to identify his body. My late husband's funeral was a very small, brief gathering where I had prerecorded Bible verses and prayers.

The coffin was decorated with the flag of Grenada and, because Trevor was a James Bond fan who loved playing with Lego with his children, an Aston Martin automobile made from Lego that his sons crafted. In a West African tradition, we cut up a piece of African cloth, placed one piece in the coffin, and shared other pieces with Trevor's family and funeral participants, establishing an enduring connection between Trevor and his survivors.

And then the burial—the cemetery only allowed one person onto the premises. So I stood there with my pastor on FaceTime and I flipped the camera so he could do the committal. I had to stand at my husband's grave alone, barely able to stand because I contracted COVID taking care of him. That's what a COVID burial was like. And the grief. It was incomprehensible and surreal.

The Cornerstone Baptist Church, Bergen Beach Youth Organization, Veronica's former students, members of the Fletcher children's school community, and her children's former soccer coaches participated in a motorcade in Trevor's honor organized by the children's godmother.

We stood outside our home and they circled the block several times in their cars with signs. They blew the horn and told us how much they loved us. One of the deacons from my church prayed for us on a megaphone. Neighbors came out onto their porches. That was the closest anyone could get to us because of COVID.

Afterward people did drive-bys and brought food for us. Other than that, we were completely isolated and alone.

Over time, youth Bible study at Cornerstone Baptist Church, enrollment in a local culinary school, the Boy Scouts and the Girl Scouts, church activities, and extracurricular activities at school helped the Fletcher children, Joshua, Zachary, and Madison, cope with their father's death.

At a point in time when it was safer to gather outside, Trevor's transit brothers and sisters from the Flatbush Depot sanitized a bus and sanitized his work tools. And they drove a big city bus to our house and brought his tools home.

It was an honor and a privilege for these MTA brothers and sisters to come to our home and bring his toolbox home for us. And they presented us with an MTA vest. It was an honor and a privilege.

And they shared some stories about my late husband so that the children would know that we're not the only ones that missed him. He wasn't only important to us, he was important to other people, too. And when I did a graduation party for my sons, transit employees came to the party, just to tell the kids, "Congratulations. We're proud of you."

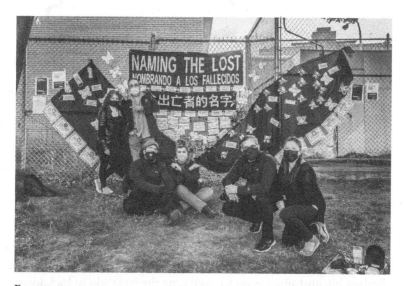

FIGURE 9

As COVID deaths mounted, the artists, activists, and folklorists of Naming the Lost Memorials created sites of mourning across New York City, using the languages of surrounding neighborhoods. This one was at Jacobi Medical Center in the Bronx, where sirens sounded constantly during the worst days of COVID. Back left to front right: Elena Martínez, Bobby Sanabria, Luis Pagán, Leenda Bonilla, Edl Alvarez, and Martha Zarate. Photograph by Erik McGregor for Naming the Lost Memorials, City Lore Archive.

5

Coping, Spring 2020

When New Yorkers confronted the pandemic, some bravely faced danger to serve the public. A few pretended there was no reason to change their daily routines. The rest of us endured, finding big and small ways to overcome the isolation of lockdown, connect with others, and maybe even reduce the suffering of friends, family, and neighbors.

The goal in the spring of 2020 was to "flatten the curve,"[1] or slow the spread of the infection. Closing businesses, houses of worship, and schools, and urging everyone to stay home, gave the virus fewer opportunities to spread from one person to another; with a reduced spread, hospitals would receive fewer patients and could better care for those who came in their doors—an urgent imperative when hospitals were overflowing and hundreds were dying each day.

In their efforts to cope in an uncertain time, many found stability and strength in the daily television briefings of Governor Cuomo, who combined a tough yet humane demeanor with a commitment to relying on facts when making decisions.[2]

For many in the city and state of New York, and nationwide, Cuomo was a reliable source of information and a steadying leader, particularly in comparison to the erratic President Trump, and to Mayor de Blasio, who underplayed the danger of the virus, disagreed with his own health department, and acted slowly in response to COVID-19. But Cuomo had flaws as well. His ongoing quarrels with Mayor de Blasio delayed city and state action. And as early as March 2020, Cuomo's administration directed nursing homes to accept elderly COVID-19 patients who were discharged from hospitals, then undercounted the surge in deaths that followed and worked to conceal their full extent.[3]

If Cuomo helped the general public cope, countless individuals found their own ways to deal with the pandemic, helping immediate friends and family, or working to build collective strength in a badly shaken city.

In a time when close contact carried the threat of infection, one coping strategy was to huddle up—as a couple, a family, or mixture of friends and family—to ride out the pandemic in a residential group, or "pod." Exchanging the wider world for the support of a small circle of roommates, such New Yorkers learned to highlight their weeks with everything from dinners to dance sessions to workouts to binging on television.

When so much seemed unstable, enduring sources of belief became important. Firmly religious people could double down on their faith because it offered hope in desperate circumstances. Secular and religious New Yorkers alike looked beyond the present and envisioned a fairer and healthier future that would redeem the sufferings and inequalities of 2020.

As long days of isolation dulled the senses, beauty, too, became more important. As the spring advanced, people could be seen gazing with wonder at flowers that blossomed in the patches of earth surrounding street trees. Some photographed the blooms with cell phones and posted them online, sharing signs of life in the midst of death and spreading beautiful images in a visually parched city.

Social media helped people connect online. Zoom became a way of gathering for religious services, lectures, meetings, concerts, conversations, parties, and oral history interviews. New Yorkers who left the city for country houses (and discovered that the fears bred by the pandemic followed them) used social media to maintain contact with friends and relatives in the city. Teachers used various platforms (with mixed results) to teach classes.

Nightly cheers for essential workers provided an opportunity for connection, but the city was not as one. Some New Yorkers denied the dangers of COVID-19 or scorned masks and social distancing. Heavy-breathing joggers who passed near pedestrians drew scorn. In southern Brooklyn many Orthodox Jews rejected masking and social distancing because they wanted to continue religious and cultural traditions at all costs. Governor Cuomo and Mayor de Blasio criticized police for not adhering to masking requirements.[4] Even more troubling, some New Yorkers blamed Asian Americans for the virus. The actions of President Trump—who had repeatedly referred to COVID-19 as the "Chinese virus" despite warnings that this would set off racist reactions—echoed into New York City and shaped everyday life under COVID-19. Asian Americans suffered attacks ranging from slurs to physical assaults.[5]

In the spring of 2020, there were definitely heroes—people who knew the dangers of COVID-19 and risked their lives to help others in need. More of us got by on something less exalted, but still important: a dogged adherence to the demands of social distancing. Whether you stayed at home in the city to avoid getting infected or left town, the practical result was the same: fewer people getting sick, and fewer patients in hard-pressed hospitals. The Chinese American folklorist Mackenzie Kwok got at this when she wrote, "As New Yorkers are well aware, life goes on not because we are brave, but because we have no other choice."[6]

By the end of May 2020, New York City's tally of infections, hospitalizations, and deaths showed that the city's collective efforts to "flatten the curve" of COVID-19 had succeeded. On May 26, the number of deaths was down to sixty-one per day—a fraction of the almost eight hundred per day calculated on April 11. This was a collective victory that New Yorkers could be proud of.[7]

With the decline in infections and deaths, the rationale for keeping New York on PAUSE would be open to question. But in a city where people had coped with the pandemic in so many different ways—from sheltering at home to working on the frontlines, from vigilant masking to skepticism about masking—it was not clear what kind of city would appear when New York emerged from lockdown.

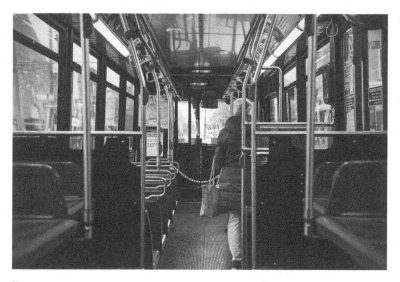

FIGURE 10
March 28, 2020: Bus configured to keep passengers away from the bus operator. Photograph by Megan Green.

Davidson Garrett

Davidson Garrett, a poet, writer, and actor who lives on East 28th Street in Manhattan, drove a taxi in New York City from 1978 to 2018. His poem first appeared in Coronavirus Haiku, edited by Mark Nowak for the Worker Writers School.[8]

no opera now
the virus darkened the Met
but birds sing to me

Embracing Solitude

Adele Dressner

Shortly before the pandemic began, Adele Dressner, who lives on the Upper East Side of Manhattan, lost her partner and retired after serving for forty years as president of All-In-One Suppliers, a store fixture and display business founded by her uncle Herman Dressner in 1914.[9]

ON MARCH 11, 2020, I celebrated my birthday with my nephew, niece, and two great nieces. We met in a Korean restaurant, washed our hands (since we were somewhat aware that something troublesome was on the New York horizon), and shared food and laughter. We tentatively hugged goodbye, and I hopped on the Q train to ride four stops back to my home.

It was a great evening. The very next day, I received a call from my niece who told me that her brother (the nephew who dined with us the night before) was very sick with COVID and that I should not even think about leaving my apartment for the foreseeable future. I have been there ever since.

What I have learned is that I can be alone, something I always dreaded. I have lost two long-term loves in my life, and each time I was devastated, and only was able to resume some semblance of normalcy because of the support and love of friends and family who made sure that I was never alone if I didn't want to be.

I have also learned that in solitude there can be growth. When you are more focused, and not busy with an over-scheduled life, it does allow for more introspection. I almost never cooked in these past years (with or without my special person by my side) but preferred to dine out with friends, enjoying the social aspects as well as sampling new cuisine. Now I prepare healthy and, to my surprise, very creative meals for myself. Full disclosure: I would rather be sharing something I made with someone I love, but since that is not prudent at this time, I have learned to adapt and even enjoy the experience.

I have personally known several Holocaust survivors, and have always been deeply interested, actually fascinated, by their stories. I found out that one thing they all had in common, was an ability to live one day, actually one minute at a time, and not think about

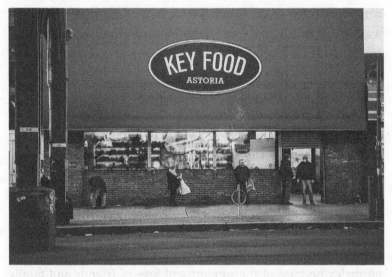

FIGURE 11

April 10, 2020: Social distancing outside a supermarket in Astoria, Queens. Photograph by Megan Green. She wrote: "I'm a professional photographer and also work an overnight graphics gig (which I am grateful to be able to do from home), so I'm awake at odd hours. To avoid exposure I take early morning walks to twenty-four-hour stores to buy what I need when the rest of the world is asleep. I started taking pictures of all of the signs in the storefronts to document the little pockets of early morning activity on the otherwise empty streets. This is an ongoing project for me now—I stay in as much as possible—but when I go on a grocery run I'll take the long way to take photos."

the future. I am trying, albeit not always successfully, to follow that example, and to have some hope that life will resume in some way, and that we will all prevail.

I try not to dwell on the fact that so many people have succumbed to the coronavirus, but to look instead to a future that will be worthwhile for all. I have always cared about social justice and have volunteered in many arenas. This situation has only increased that interest and commitment in me. Being idle, and not having a purpose in life, is at best an empty existence. I always knew this but being forced into solitude has made me more focused on doing more for others.

I have seen that adversity brings out the best and worst in people. Friends and family who I did not hear from regularly are now checking in much more often, but conversely, I have observed that some people who you thought would be there, are not. I try not to judge, but I cannot help but observe. It seems that for some, friendship is more about what you do together, rather than what you feel for each other. For the most part, however, I am very happy to report that in my case, I have received a great deal of love and concern from all my family (some of whom were too busy to keep in touch very often in normal times) and neighbors as well as friends. I have also become more aware that everyone handles adversity in different ways. I always knew this, but now I feel it as well.

A Prayer for My Mother

Sumya Abida

Sumya Abida, from the Soundview section of the Bronx, grew up in a Bangladeshi family. Although religion was not a part of her own life, she found a route to prayer when COVID-19 threatened her mother, who worked as a nurse in a Bronx hospital. In March 2020, while she was a student at Bard High School Early College in Manhattan, she wrote this journal entry as part of an assignment.[10]

Entry 1: A Dua For My Mother
I am not religious.
I don't have the best relationship with my mother.
But in the darkness of our reality today, I need to find light.
Through Allah, for my mother.

Today my mother comes home from work. My father is in the living room watching the daily news informing of another thousand lives lost to the coronavirus in New York. It is 4:30 p.m. and I am taking a nap in my room. My mother walks in and like any other day she reminds me to do my afternoon prayer. And as usual, I find a way to get out of it. Right now, I want to sleep some more so I quietly wait for her to leave the room. But after a quick peek from beneath my blanket, I see her still there. She is looking at herself in the mirror next to my bed. Ten minutes pass and my mother is still there, gazing at her reflection. I wonder, what could she have been thinking about in those ten minutes?

Little did I realize that while I was grumbling about wanting to sleep a few extra minutes, my mother was trembling in fear. Filled with relentless anxiety, she looks at herself in the mirror, not smiling, but holding back many, many tears. They were the kinds of tears she didn't want anyone at home to wonder about because then she must face the difficult task: how do you tell your children "There is a chance I might not return home one day"?

My mother is a nurse at a hospital in the Bronx. She works a 7–4 shift five days a week. Some days she'll work a double shift to make the extra money since my father no longer works, and she's the only one supporting our family with a stable income. Recently, there has been a higher call for people working at her hospital to do extra hours but I wish she didn't have to go to work at all. There is no certainty for her health and survival in the work she is constantly involving herself in. How safe even is the space for her? Is she wearing an N95 mask at all times? Does she have enough PPE on? Can she breathe?

The closest I can get to any of these answers are through our few and brief workday phone calls. But those have been the hardest conversations to hear when she is literally telling me, in Bengali:

"I want to quit so badly. It's frightening working here. My life is always on the line when I interact with another patient who tests positive for the coronavirus. I am scared, Sumya, but I can't just quit or else our family will suffer. Please do your *namaz* [a prayer] and make *dua* [a wish delivered in the context of a prayer] for me and our family . . ."

On her side of the telephone line, she hears "Ok. I will. Yes, ma. Ok."

With every demoralizing, single-syllable word of guilt that rolls down my tongue, another tear rolls down my mother's cheek. When I can't speak fluent Bengali and she can't speak fluent English, how do I communicate my sincerest feelings to her? How do I tell my mother, "Please quit, ma. Write a resignation letter before it's too late. I need you. I need you here with me."

The sound of her voice is growing weaker. Yet, she continues to walk through my bedroom door as I take another afternoon nap, in hopes of receiving my prayers. How selfish could I have been? She is shaking in terror and I am sleeping. She is fighting on the frontlines of a global pandemic and I am sleeping. She is begging me to pray for her goddamn survival and I am sleeping.

It's true, we've never had a lovely, stable relationship. Our relationship is one filled with betrayal, unresolved misunderstandings, many silent treatments, and a lack of trust. But right now, we are no longer in a situation where I can be comfortable in the grudges I held against her. She is still my mother. And right now, my mother needs me and I need her more than ever. I don't know how to say "I love you" to her but if there is one thing I can do for my mother, it is to call for Allah in her name.

Today I will pray with intention, for the sake of my mother who is fighting at risk every day for a world beyond herself.

Thus I offer a dua for my mother and a portion of my own prayers:

One who recites Ayatul Kursi seeks a blessing from Allah for protection. When one leaves home and recites Ayatul Kursi, Allah sends a group of angels to come and protect them from any harm.

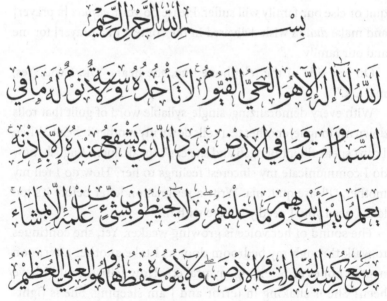

FIGURE 12
Ayatul Kursi in Arabic. Photograph by Ridwan Taufik / Shutterstock.

Transliteration of Ayatul Kursi: Allahu laaa ilaaha illaa huwal haiyul qai-yoom; laa taakhuzuhoo sinatunw wa laa nawm; lahoo maa fissamaawaati wa maa fil ard; man zallazee yashfa'u indahooo illaa be iznih; ya'lamu maa baina aideehim wa maa khalfahum; wa laa yuheetoona beshai 'immin 'ilmihee illa be maa shaaaa; wasi'a kursiyyuhus samaa waati wal arda wa la ya'ooduho hifzuhumaa; wa huwal aliyyul 'azeem.

And here is a portion of my own prayer.

Allah,

It's Sumya. Can you hear me? It's a new voice calling for you today. I know I'm not a devout Muslim and I also know this is my first time truly praying since . . . uh, I don't even know. But I come to you today with the purest of intentions, seeking for you to hear my prayers and grant my sincerest wishes. It's for my mother, Anowara Begum. You recognize that name, right? She's one amongst many of your most faithful believers. She's also a hero on Earth. But being the hero in a blue uniform and an N95 mask, her own life is also at risk. You know why, right? I don't mean to request something so grand of you as to eradicate a whole pandemic overnight, I simply wish for you to look out for my mother. Keep her safe while she's working in the hospital, please? Wherever my mother is, will you watch over her from above? I come to you today daring to ask for your help after all the wrong I've done to my mother over the years. But for her life, will you forgive me this once? Will you hear me just this once, Allah?

With sincere wishes,

Sumya

Sharing Stories

Matilda Virgilio Clark

Matilda Virgilio Clark found strength and pleasure in recounting her family's history for younger generations. Born in Italy, she immigrated to the United States and lived in New York City and Long Island before settling in Dobbs Ferry, New York. She worked as a seamstress, babysitter, house cleaner, and administrative assistant, earned a BA in sociology and business at Molloy College, and served as a life coach.[11]

DURING THIS TIME of reflection in isolation, I had the chance to lower the volume of all the noise that normally accompanies my day to day and find a new center. I discovered the wonder of connecting with grandchildren and family on Zoom meetings and rediscovered my love of writing bits and pieces of the untold stories of our family's years in Italy. Previously no one in my family was interested, but now that they are all homebound and far away, suddenly memories have value.

I write several times a week on our shared Facebook family page, and it has encouraged others in the family to also post. I told stories about my grandfather who went back and forth between Italy and the United States before World War I: he worked as a cowboy, a mason, and a railroad worker. He struck gold (and later lost it) in the Klondike Gold Rush before traveling to New York to work on the subway. I told them about my own steerage-class journey to American with my mother and brother in November 1954—two trunks, two suitcases, and $200 on a voyage that made us seasick. I was six years old, but I was sustained by my mother's words when we left Italy: "Whatever happens, God is with us."

When I tell these stories it feels like Sunday around the table over pasta again, a tradition that was lost after Mamma died and the children moved out of state.

Isolation rekindled my desire to share the stories and the new generation's desire to hear them. We are an immigrant family with memories of hard work, learning a new language, and adapting to cold weather after growing up in the sunshine of southern Italy. Much has been sacrificed so that the young would benefit. To ignore that felt disrespectful to the memory of all who brought us to this day.

Even if there are daily struggles to stay healthy, get provisions, and manage our finances, the groundwork was set by those before us. Our family is prepared for the challenge to survive and is able to face adversity with energy, hope, and perseverance. These are the qualities that have been taught and continue to be passed on to the newborn.

I am glad to report back to the ancestors long gone that we have carried on their work with dignity and valor. Their efforts and sacrifices were not in vain.

I am the last of the elders with all the stories. I now have the luxury of time to document them as best I can to pass them on to the generations yet to be.

A Subway Story in the Time of COVID-19

Ron Kolm

Ron Kolm is a poet and long-time resident of Long Island City, Queens. He saw his fifty-year career in bookstores terminated by the pandemic and was on unemployment when a journey into Manhattan presented him with an opportunity to help save a life.[12]

I had to travel into Manhattan
to cash my unemployment check,
so I sat in the front car, wearing
a mask, doing my best
to avoid the other passengers.
After leaving the bank
I walked back to Union Square station
and found a place on the platform
where there weren't too many people
standing around waiting.

Time goes by and no train appears.
There's a sudden movement
as a woman, maybe late 50s,
tosses her bag and her mask onto the tracks,
then clumsily climbs down
and joins them.
"Hey, what's up?" I shout through my mask.
She moans and says
that this is how she's going to get home,
she's tired of everything.

She edges over towards the third rail,
and unfortunately
because my back is so messed up
I can't physically grab her
so I unleash my best zinger:

"Do you believe in any kind of God?
Because if you do, you gotta know
how pissed off he or she's gonna be
if you touch that thing!"

A young guy
comes running over,
jumps onto the tracks
and lifts the lady up,
depositing her on the platform.
He holds her
waiting for the police,
who do show up pretty quickly.
My train finally arrives, and I go home,
amazed at how the Universe works.

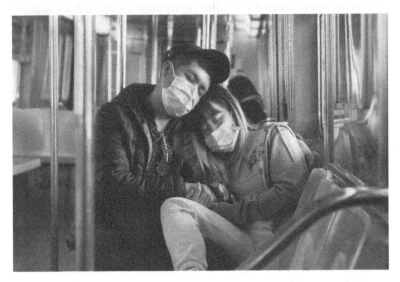

FIGURE 13
Aboard the Queens-bound R train, April 2020: affection, exhaustion, and masking. Photograph by Josue Tepancal Jimenez.

Making Masks, Whatever It Takes

Lily M. Chin

Lily M. Chin of Greenwich Village, a knit and crochet designer and instructor, was jolted into mask making by the spring surge of 2020.[13]

I KNEW SEVERAL friends, associates, who died of COVID. Others survived but still live with the medical consequences like needing a walker and still requiring an oxygen tank.

Ten blocks from me, a major health facility had the dreaded and necessary refrigerated trucks for the bodies. I'd pass by it on evening walks and veer away.

I have good friends and family who are doctors and nurses. My cousin and her husband are both health care providers and she quit so as not to leave their children orphaned should both of them fall to the disease.

It's not hyperbole to say I felt scared and helpless. I felt a need to do SOMEthing, but didn't know what. Masks were scarce. The N95s were discouraged for "civilians" as even the health pros didn't have enough. But production for masks for everyone else had not ramped up yet. Thus, those with do-it-yourself skills were at an advantage.

I joined groups online about mask making as my seamstress skills are woefully lacking. I had a "real" sewing machine that saw very little action as well as a couple of "toys," plastic jobbies that did rudimentary stuff. I printed out scads of models from the standard surgical to my favorite, the "duck bill." However, as a person with a science background [Chem major in college, pre-med track] I knew that cloth, even doubled, has its limitations.

So off I went into the rabbit hole of do-it-yourself science groups doing everything from mechanizing manual ventilators to jerry rigging face shields with 3-D printing. I found that surgical wrapping material for sterilizing instruments in hospitals, when doubled, had extraordinary efficacy on par with N95's (though it doesn't have the tight fit that fit testing ensures). I got my wonderful dentist to use his dental license to order some up from a medical supply company!

I also found filters, Blue Shop towels, and other highly effective alternatives. In a nutshell, much better than the standard woven fabrics. Now for the making.

I sewed and sewed until my real machine broke down. I went to both my toy alternatives until they broke down. None of the repair shops here in New York were open as they were deemed nonessential. I resorted to sewing by hand.

I ran out of elastic and found elastic online was as scarce as flour and sour dough starters. I took some off old underwear. I cut up old T-shirts. I even used Cascade Yarns' "Fixation" cotton with spandex. Whatever it took.

I made more than five hundred masks and gave them away for free to local hospitals and hospital workers, the essential workers, the homeless out in the street, friends, neighbors . . . I just wanted everyone around me to be safe. Selfishly, I wanted everyone around me to be less infectious.

We're in a much better place now. New York's positivity rate is less than half a percent and we're close to a 70 percent vaccination rate.

I've yet to get my sewing machines fixed but intend to do so soon.

Working and Surviving

Kleber Vera (Flame)

Kleber Vera, a hairstylist and LGBT activist living in Jackson Heights, Queens, performed in drag as Flame, worked with the AIDS Center of Queens County, and read stories to children throughout New York City at libraries, schools, open street events, and cultural centers. Unemployed and isolated in the early months of the pandemic, they found new work designing wigs and making masks.[14]

I SPENT A lot of time at home just watching the news and trying to stay really attentive and find out what is going on here. And it was really tense after that. I actually put myself into self-quarantine for the first three months of it. So it was a really scary time because nobody really knew what was going on, except that there was something serious, dangerous, and potentially deadly going around. It was very scary.

The salons all closed down. I had a few clients reach out to me that wanted to get their hair done. But honestly I was so scared and nervous I refused to take on clients. I put myself in self-quarantine and I just didn't feel comfortable or safe seeing anybody.

I wasn't working, I wasn't making any income and I was eating through my savings. And then the first three months of lockdown, I had to dip into my savings to pay the bills, mortgage maintenance, everything else.

I live in Jackson Heights, just a few blocks from Elmhurst Hospital. In the first three months of lockdown all I could hear out my window, literally 24/7, was the sirens of the ambulances coming off the BQE going into the hospital. So it's been really, really intense for me.

As far as the streets, I remember I would only go outside to go food shopping, and you definitely noticed a vibe of just tension in the air. People were very scared. People were trying to avoid each other, but at the same time, like sometimes fighting over certain products that they wanted to buy. I saw an incident where this lady didn't want to wear a mask and the manager was called and she's coughing on people, and she was asked to leave and it was just crazy.

I spent a couple of thousand dollars panic buying like a lot of people were doing at the time, buying food, canned foods, toilet paper, all that stuff. I ate through my savings very, very quickly within that first three months of lockdown. And then after that, there was still no income being made. So it's been a huge, huge struggle.

It's been really stressful on my family. My mother and my step-father are seniors. So I've been really careful about not seeing them. I used to see my family once a week. They live in Yonkers, and I would visit every weekend to spend time with my mom and my siblings and other immediate family. And that's completely changed.

I've been up to Yonkers, maybe two or three times in the last year instead of every week.

I actually had a few family members pass away: two family members passed away from it in Ecuador, elderly family members. And that was obviously stressful. I've seen my friends on my Facebook feed posts. Some of them knew several people, nine, ten, eleven, twelve people that got COVID or that passed away.

My friends definitely have had it. I might have had it as well. I tested positive for the antibodies. Luckily my health wasn't too affected by that, but it's really hard for me to hear people that still deny it and think that it's not real. I've seen it. I've felt it, I've lived it.

In the beginning of the pandemic, the first three months or so of lockdown, I got really, really depressed, and I wasn't doing much because my life went from being so, so busy to just sitting around wondering, 'Oh my God, what's going to happen next?' To keep myself mentally occupied and stimulated, I started working on my craft.

Since I couldn't do hair in the salon anymore, I started working on wigs, designing wigs and selling them online to try to make a little extra money. I started making my own masks, with a little special flair and design. I like to think I have a pretty unique style. I had fun making masks, selling those online to try to make a little money. I started doing weekly Facebook live events where I would just go on live and just try to talk to people about self-care and try to stay in touch with my friends that way, find out what people were doing.

Sustaining Community

Sheikh Musa Drammeh

When COVID-19 restrictions prevented Muslim worshippers from gathering in person, Sheikh Musa Drammeh worked to provide alternative ways of meeting. Born in the Gambia in 1962, he immigrated to New York City in 1986. A longtime educator and community activist in the Parkchester section of the Bronx, he is the founder of the Islamic Leadership School and the Muslim Media Corporation, the publisher of the Muslim Community Report, New York Parrot, *and* Parkchester Times *newspapers, and CEO of Halalfinder.com.*[15]

THIS RAMADAN WAS the most challenging that we've ever experienced. Ramadan is the month of getting together, eating together, fellowship, hospitality, and neighborliness. And these all involve coming together physically. Unfortunately this year we couldn't do any of those activities. Everything was canceled. Even the mosques were closed. It was a month that we pray will never ever be repeated.

People could not pray in congregational prayer. Everything was done individually, and it was very, very painful. And it was confusing to some people. But because of the adaptability of human beings, we were able to adopt the virtual platform to continue on with the spirit of fasting.

We adapted and we're still learning how to get our messages effectively to these virtual platforms.

Years before COVID-19 struck, Sheikh Drammeh engaged in community projects with neighborhood Jews and loaned a Jewish congregation space in his mosque.

One of the benefits of living in a place like New York is the availability of so many useful tools and resources. The government quickly put together places where people can go and get their halal and kosher meals. So that even though they cannot attend mosque or synagogue to eat together, they can carry it home. That was very, very helpful. Even some of the families that could not leave their homes, they were able to get their meals. The city hired cab drivers to deliver these meals. So we are very, very grateful to the innovativeness of the city. Much as it was painful not coming together, the inventiveness of the city made it easier to manage. That's number one.

People of all backgrounds came together.

Number two, New Yorkers of all backgrounds came together as neighbors. I have never experienced such neighborliness—calling neighbors, especially the seniors and the disabled and the widows, to find out if there's a need for laundry assistance, to provide medical delivery, or if there's a need to provide shopping assistance, due to the pandemic situation.

So, you know, it's a tragedy. We lost a lot of people. But I firmly believe that the tragedy will leave us to be better human beings, stronger societies. Once in a while it takes a tragedy to understand that there's a symbiotic relationship among residents, regardless of ethnicity, where they come from. We are in it together. And this pandemic has shown us that we have to be together.

One of the most painful realities of COVID-19 is having your uncle, or your father, or your spouse, lying by him- or herself and no loved one can come to the bedside, to talk and comfort and read whatever reading that is. That is something that is almost as painful as death because in your last moments there are customs within the Muslim community, where you sit right next to them and comfort them, you pray for them. And you remind them of the fact that this is the last moment, they have their place, and you reading Quran and the verses will remind them of that.

And unfortunately there were some Muslims that could not get a proper Islamic burial. That was absolutely atrocious, to have a family member that you couldn't see in his or her final days, and you couldn't bury properly.

We have lost so many people in the African community. One ethnic group alone, the Fulani community, lost over forty family members and now I'm sure that number, has either doubled or tripled. And that's just one ethnic group in the African Muslim community.

The Bengali community is one of the hardest hit immigrant communities in New York City. They've lost so many people, including some of the most well-known Bengali Muslim leaders.

We did not manage it well. We just went through it. But anybody that tells you the management was properly done did not know what they're talking about. It was just the best we can, but the pain and the suffering still lingers.

We are communal beings.

As a member of the Muslim community and the African community, regardless of what religion, we are communal beings. We are not individualistic people. We are part of a larger community, regardless of race or ethnicity. We are part of this strong community that will come together to fend for our loved ones. Those who are dying feel some type of comfort knowing that since they were part of a larger community, their loved ones will be taken care of after their departure.

In the Muslim community, the Prophet said God never sent a disease or sickness without sending the remedy for it. Even though we currently do not have a remedy for COVID-19, we firmly believe that the remedy is there someplace. And we believe that one day scientists will discover it. So COVID-19 has claimed so many lives worldwide, but the remedy is coming. That is our firm belief as a religious people.

So many traditional remedies, traditional methods of mitigating pain we use in Africa and other places are being used—warm water with lemon and ginger and honey blocks. Additionally, we're still using prayers and we're still following hand hygiene, and still wearing our mask, but other than that, nothing else. We're still keeping hope alive, knowing that very soon, by the mercy of God, scientists will discover remedies. So that's where we are with COVID-19.

This pandemic had some bright spotlight on the painful disparities, economic health disparities, wealth disparities, educational disparities, environmental disparities. When we look at the victims of COVID-19, most of the deaths are occurring within the Latino and African American communities and Native Americans. I call it a crime.

In October 2020, Sheikh Drammeh launched a campaign to push for equitable public health policies and encourage people to take more responsibility for their health by eating right and getting exercise.

The misleading messengers are always active, you know, politically, spiritually, socially, educationally. They hijack the narrative, mislead people and lead them to their destruction. During this pandemic, no difference. Unfortunately, what makes it even worse is that you know it was coming from the top of our government, from the president down, promoting this nonsense.

Muslim leaders neutralized misleading information.

But what we did early on, especially the Muslim community, is that Muslim leaders came together so very quickly, and then brought rules to be followed, including adhering to the social distancing rules. Including wearing mask, including disassociating the pandemic from religious practices, everything.

And there were hundreds of Muslim and African leaders teaching the same thing. And that has made a huge difference. The misleading noises were neutralized by individuals like me and hundreds of other imams and African leaders. So we are very grateful that we took this issue head on, so that whatever coming from the White House or anywhere else will be neutralized before they infest our community. So until today, people listen to us more than they listen to the misleading elements in our society. And we are grateful.

Building Bonds

Keerthan Thiyagarajah

Keerthan Thiyagarajah, a cook and a student, took strength from his neighborhood of Jackson Heights, Queens, the home of many immigrants.[16]

I THINK THE biggest changes in my life personally are school. Being a culinary management student, you have to be there in person to learn.

I think relationships grew a lot closer. That was one of the ups, I guess, of this pandemic. I think I learned to love a lot more and care about the people around me.

Being Asian it's hard enough, but with the pandemic on top of it, it's like an added weight to our shoulders. And I think because of politics and the news and whatnot, we're looked at as second-class people. And it's been tough, but I think we've gotten through, and we've learned, and I especially learned to love and care about people more and the ones around me.

Everybody looks out for each other. My community is very tight, even though we're not all the same color. We're not all the same ethnicities. We all care for each other.

I grew up in this area, Jackson Heights. I was born at Elmhurst Hospital. This is my neighborhood. This is where I remember all my childhood memories coming from. This is the melting pot of Queens. When you think of Queens, you go to Jackson Heights, you have every single piece of food. You want every piece of culture, you get it there. And seeing it just disappear in a matter of days was nerve wracking, especially 74th and Roosevelt.

There's traffic there all the time. These streets are flooded all the time. And just to see it completely disappear was crazy. To see it go away within like weeks and days, it was something new.

And then seeing my childhood hospital being overrun by the pandemic, watching this hospital that I grew up at being overrun to the point where they had to store bodies in the back of ice trucks. And in the back of the hospital, there are just lines of trucks of deceased people from COVID-19. And there's nothing you can do about it. There's no room for disposing of a body properly. And they would just throw them in the back of a truck and that was it.

People are not on the streets anymore, there's no traffic, there's no honking, there's not anything. Stores are boarded up with wood because of a possibility of ransacking. That was a major thing. People were scared of their livelihood being taken away from them. It was something out of a movie, like *The Walking Dead* or something. It was scary to see all of this unfold.

No one in this community is rich. This community is middle-class people working hard. Most of them first generation, people coming in from all across the world, coming into Jackson Heights and hoping to make a livelihood whether it's driving a taxi, or opening up a food stand.

The biggest need in the community was someone to look up to. And I don't think we had that. That's why there was a lot of people dying in this area.

I think a leader was someone that we needed most. That didn't happen.

Jackson Heights is one of those places where there's a bond between everybody and whether you're Black, White, blue, gold, it doesn't matter what you are. There's always a bond in that neighborhood. And whether you need help, you can just ask for it and someone will with open arms, help you. In anything you need.

Organizing

Dave Crenshaw

Dave Crenshaw, a coach and community organizer, grew up in a family of African American activists in southern Washington Heights. In the 1980s, when violence surrounding the crack trade scarred his neighborhood, he worked to give young people alternatives to dangerous streets. He went on to found the Uptown Team Dreamers, a program based at PS 128 that was devoted to sports, community service, and education that welcomed beginner athletes and girls. His work earned him the nickname Coach Dave. During the COVID-19 pandemic he worked with longstanding allies to provide food, masks, testing, and eventually vaccinations in Washington Heights.[17]

WHEN THIS THING hit I lost a lot of people. I lost my brother—not to COVID but to COVID circumstances. I lost my uncle, I lost my cousin. I lost a super and his wife. And one that hit me really hard was when I lost my best friend from high school, Reverend Craig Woods. And I never even got a chance to hear him preach.

And at that moment, I knew I could not hibernate. I knew I had to stay out there. My neighborhood was counting on me.

Crenshaw put on an N95 mask and went out to deliver food to people. Over the course of the pandemic, his partners included the Uptown Dreamers, the Community League of the Heights (CLOTH), Black Health, the Northern Manhattan Improvement Corporation, the bookstore Word Up, the Dominican American public servant Maria Luna, and Dean Robert Fullilove and his students at Columbia University's Mailman School of Public Health.

The blue mask is not bad, but the 95 keeps you alive. That was my philosophy.

I teamed up with CLOTH to get food to the seniors. Instead of doing a food pantry twice a week, they went to four, five days, and longer hours. And the line used to go from 159th all the way down to 158th. That's how long the line was every day.

But then you have seniors who couldn't get food. So I was helping deliver food to the seniors—one of my best workouts, because I think they gave me every apartment building that had no elevator.

My idea was I had to put people at ease, let them know we're going to stick together. Food became a very important tool to give out. Even when the food was given to us cold, we would heat it up, put the barbecue sauce on it, roll around the neighborhood and give it to the ones that didn't go to soup kitchens and food pantries.

If walkup buildings were an obstacle for food deliveries, the use of masks was complicated by mixed messaging from authorities on the value of masking and residents' reluctance to wear masks.

It took forever just to get people to wear masks. People really did not want to mask in the beginning. They just couldn't understand the importance of it. And there was a lot of misinformation going out. Some people tried to do everything. Some people said, "I'm not doing nothing." Some people were wiping down everything they could wipe down. And some said, "Don't believe this. I'm not wiping down nothing."

The information was coming from so many different places. So wild and crazy. Even the CDC was not dependable. You couldn't count on them, they would send out multiple messages. I do know Dr. Fauci had the hardest job in the world, trying to deliver information.

By the time the testing was widespread, we had developed a good relationship with the community, because we'd been giving out masks, and we'd been helping people get food supplies, and we'd been giving out books. With Word Up bookstore, we started getting books. Parents were staying on line for an hour or two. What did the kids get out of it? We got them books. The sad thing is that some families didn't want books, but the families that did were very happy.

And we just had to explain the importance of testing, helping people figure out how to get appointments. Everything we did, technology was a barrier.

You had to talk with people, you had to convince them, you had to treat them correctly so they don't just walk away. That's what the hardest part was. And at the testing sites we were also giving out masks and information. We were giving out hand sanitizer. We became like little walk-in, pop-up clinics, going to different areas at different times.

Sometimes people needed an incentive to get tested.

Same thing with HIV. Same thing with AIDS. We don't want to deal with it. Avoidance. Nobody wants to get the bad news. The biggest thing we had to explain to people was you can get it and have no symptoms.

We were not forcing anyone to do anything. That was not my job. My role was: those of you who want to hear this, those who want access, this is where you can go. After a while, we became the masters at just telling people where everything was at.

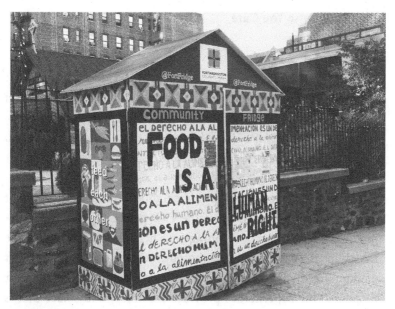

FIGURE 14

New Yorkers established mutual aid projects not in a spirit of charity, but of people helping one another cope with the hardships of the pandemic. Among the most visible were community refrigerators, like this one in Washington Heights, where residents left food for neighbors. Photograph by James Melchiorre.

Clap Because You Care

Led Black

On April 17, 2020, in his blog Uptown Collective *at www. uptowncollective.com, Led Black addressed a ritual that became a defining feature of the early months of the pandemic: the daily eruption of cheers, banging of pots, blasting of horns, and music at 7:00 p.m. in honor of the city's essential workers.*[18]

I THINK I SPEAK for many in this neighborhood and throughout this great city when I say that the 7:00 p.m. clapping and noise-making sessions for our courageous health care heroes on the frontlines is the highlight of the day, every day. This simple act of stopping whatever you are doing and showing appreciation for those real-life superheroes provides a comfort and solace that is hard to describe. We owe them a debt that we can never repay. The same can be said of all the "essential" workers who keep this society running and who do not have the privilege of working from home.

The timing of the daily appreciation manifestations could not be any better, as they usually start after the daily Trump propaganda briefings are over. Tyrant Trump has turned what is supposed to be a medium for crucial information on the nation's fight against the novel coronavirus into a political rally whose primary goal is the reelection of Donald Trump. Let me state this as plainly as I can, America will not survive a second term of Donald Trump.

Our lives have changed profoundly. We no longer venture outside except for necessities. The once lively Alto Manhattan is eerily and uncharacteristically quiet. When you do go out you can see the fear and despair in the eyes of your fellow New Yorkers. The gnawing uncertainty of what tomorrow will bring and the inability to meaningfully interact with one another is testing our collective sanity.

And then at 7:00 p.m., at least for a spell, we are not alone. We are united and the clouds over this city briefly part and we can see a brighter day on the horizon. The eruption of joy and togetherness provide the sustenance we all need to survive the pandemic. We are truly all in this together.

Great nations need exceptional leadership in times of crisis. We don't have that at the federal level where it is so badly needed. The American Experiment is in trouble. This is an existential crisis that goes beyond health care. The novel coronavirus is brutally exposing what has become of a once-great country. God help us all!

Pa'lante Siempre Pa'lante!

6

Opening Up, Summer and Fall 2020

As May 2020 drew to a close, and the number of deaths from COVID-19 slid downward in New York City, elected officials anticipated a gradual and methodical reopening. Instead, the city was jolted back to life by demonstrations in response to the death of George Floyd, a Black man, at the hands of Minneapolis police on May 25. Floyd's excruciating death, the life choked out of him by an officer's knee pressed into the back of his neck for some nine minutes, was captured on a bystander's cell phone. The video went viral, and protests erupted nationwide. The first recorded demonstration in New York City took place May 28, when about a hundred protesters marched from Union Square to City Hall in Manhattan. They were not the last, and similar protests flared all around the United States.

For weeks, demonstrations gripped the city. New Yorkers who took to the streets were animated not only by Floyd's death, but by echoes of earlier Black Lives Matter protests condemning the murder of Eric Garner, a Black man killed by a New York City police officer with a chokehold on Staten Island in 2014. Anger at Floyd's death was compounded by the recognition of disproportionate suffering in Black communities during the pandemic, ongoing debates over policing ("defund the police" became a prominent cry), and pent-up energy and frustration from months of lockdown.[1]

Marches, which were noticeably interracial, took the form of everything from small neighborhood gatherings to large, self-organized demonstrations that coursed through the city, drawing supporters and blocking traffic. Their mood was, by turns, angry, hopeful, and exhilarated. Most were peaceful, but when episodes of looting broke out, they renewed debates dating to the 1960s over order, justice, and the responsibilities of police and demonstrators alike. Comparisons between 2020 and 1968 were inexact, but as demonstrations mounted—and challenged police control of the streets—there was a feeling of insurrection in the air.

Since the Giuliani years in New York City, public protests had gone from being a normal part of city life to being viewed, at least from the perspective of authorities, as a nuisance that had to be controlled.[2] Yet the protests and the looting seemed to catch police off balance. Even a curfew, the first in the city since World War II, failed to halt demonstrations after dark. Aggressive police tactics for crowd control, combined with police anger over attacks on officers (both in New York and in Minneapolis, where a police station was torched), raised the temperature on city streets. Demonstrations were peaceful in Staten Island, the city's smallest and most conservative borough, but the calm that prevailed there was not evident in the rest of the city.[3]

Looters hit the posh Manhattan shopping district of Soho. A few days later they sacked mom and pop stores along ungentrified Fordham Road in the Bronx. In the Inwood section of northern Manhattan, a video recording of a police commander trying to enlist residents to prevent looting raised fears of vigilante violence. No major outbreak occurred in Inwood, but after later video footage showed local residents chasing away people presumed to be outsiders, elected officials criticized the police for playing with fire in a volatile situation.[4]

As demonstrations validated Black lives and condemned the kind of police violence that took the life of George Floyd, they also made visible, with painful clarity, deep tensions between the city's police and a significant percentage of its population.[5] Protests and debates continued through the summer over how to best police the city. Some critics called for the abolition of policing altogether, and officers—who felt insufficiently supported by city authorities— resigned from the department in record numbers. The city's Department of Investigation criticized police performance as excessive, disorganized, and indiscriminate. In 2023 the city paid more than $13 million to settle a class action lawsuit filed by protesters who said police had violated their rights.[6]

If the Black Lives Matter demonstrations of 2020 set off arguments that would last for many months, the ebbing of the first wave in the pandemic brough a decline in cases that gave residents and health workers alike a summer of rest. In spare moments, they could reflect on what they had learned and what they might do in the future. If nothing else, the demonstrations of late spring and summer suggested that large outdoor gatherings were not conducive to spreading the virus. Until October, when cases, hospitalizations, and deaths began to rise (although not in the numbers of the spring of 2020), the city regained some of its old vitality.[7]

Back in April, Governor Cuomo had mandated mask wearing when social distancing was impossible, but not until New York's lockdown was partially lifted in June were large numbers of people out and about. The return of something like a normal social life, when President Trump's hostility to masking had already politicized the issue, raised the question of how widespread masking would be received. A *New York Times* survey suggested that the practice was followed by three-quarters of New Yorkers overall.[8]

In bars and restaurants, the use of outdoor seating and curbside dining sheds helped businesses stay open but left staff with the unenviable task of having to persuade customers to wear masks when they weren't eating or drinking. This kind of burden was even greater for transit workers, who had to deal with passengers who did not want to wear masks at all. In Brooklyn in September 2020, when a bus operator repeated passengers' demands that a man coughing on a bus put on a mask, the uncooperative man knocked the bus operator unconscious. By that time, transit authorities reported, 177 transit workers—the vast majority of them bus operators—had been "harassed or assaulted" by passengers over masking and social distancing requirements.[9]

By November, cases of COVID-19 were rising in the city, bringing concerns about a new wave of infections. Staten Island, where some residents resisted masking and social distancing requirements, saw a noticeable growth in cases. When a bar owner declared his establishment an "autonomous zone" that would not comply, legal wrangling followed and battle lines were set that would last well into the future.[10]

If events in Staten Island foreshadowed future disputes at the intersection of COVID-19, public health, and politics, the presidential election of 2020 suggested new political possibilities for New York and the United States. Joe Biden handily defeated President Trump in the city; of the five boroughs Trump carried only Staten Island, long the city's most conservative borough. Protracted efforts to count absentee ballots around the United States meant that election results were not announced on the evening of Election Day, November 3. Not until November 7 did Biden gain enough electoral votes to win the presidency; when word reached

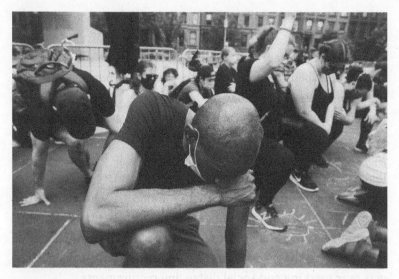

FIGURE 15
At Black Lives Matter demonstrations, protesters took a knee and recalled both Colin Kaepernick's National Football League protests against racism and the death of George Floyd, choked to death when Minneapolis police officer Derek Chauvin pressed his knee onto Floyd's neck for more than eight minutes. Photograph by Erica Lansner.

New York, the city erupted with the kind of jubilation associated with the liberation of Paris in World War II.

As 2020 came to a close in New York, vaccines against COVID-19 were being administered to medical workers and nursing home residents.[11] With a new president headed for the White House, and hope (and anxiety) in the air about the vaccine, there was reason to believe that in 2021 New York would turn some kind of corner in the pandemic.

Thomas Barzey

Thomas Barzey lives in the Bronx, where he was born and raised. Currently an actor, he has worked as a stage manager, home health aide, and office assistant. His poem first appeared in Coronavirus Haiku, edited by Mark Nowak for the Worker Writers School.[12]

New York to across Africa
Streets filled with masked protestors
Unjust killing of black lives

From Lockdown to Curfew

Clifford Pearson

In early May 2020, Clifford Pearson, a writer, urbanist, and long-time Greenwich Village resident, began a diary to record how his neighborhood functioned under the stress of the pandemic. When George Floyd died at the hands of Minneapolis police officers on May 25, Pearson's observations began to include protests in Washington Square against police violence.[13]

June 1

Just as my neighborhood was starting to emerge from two months of suspended animation and more places were reopening or preparing to test the waters, the looting began. Lily and I watched the video of George Floyd being snuffed out by a Minneapolis cop and were horrified. We followed the news reports as protesters marched in Minneapolis and then other cities. One night we saw footage of people breaking into places in downtown LA, stores and restaurants we had gone to when we lived there. The next night we heard about violence in SoHo and around Union Square, each about a mile from our apartment. Each day large groups of peaceful protesters marched through streets and into parks and squares. Yesterday evening I saw thousands head down Fifth Avenue and into Washington Square. There were speeches, chanting, sign waving, and police mostly keeping their distance. I took a few photos, then left—fearful of germs, not violence.

For the first time since 1943, New York City has a curfew. I've been here in bad times—the gritty 1980s, the Tompkins Square Park riot under Giuliani, the fallout of September 11, the blackout of 2003, the financial meltdown of 2008, and Hurricane Sandy in 2012, but never lived under curfew. This is new territory. On my way home yesterday evening, I went into Gristedes—my least favorite supermarket—and picked up some pasta sauce and canned soups, just in case. Stores that had stubbornly refused to board up their windows during the previous ten weeks as a sign of support to the neighborhood were nailing plywood to their street fronts.

Just a few days ago, all of us watched the numbers of COVID hospitalizations and deaths steadily drop and were hopeful that finally things were looking up. Most parts of New York State had entered the first phase of reopening and Cuomo said the city would probably follow suit next Monday. The early shoots of optimism may be crushed now. Is this the final blow that takes the city down?

Clueless as usual, Trump thinks that acting tough will make him look better. He threatened to use US armed forces on US citizens around the country, if governors aren't able to control their cities. It's probably an idle threat, but shocking nonetheless, a pronouncement that could push the country to the edge of martial law and a political abyss. I fear this use of the National Guard and forces in unmarked uniforms is a dry run for something bigger in November. Sure hope I'm wrong about all this.

June 2

This morning I wake up to the sounds of low-flying helicopters and sirens. When I go out for coffee I see plywood—the universal material of fear—going up on more stores and workers hammering in the nails with more urgency than yesterday. There was looting in Brooklyn and midtown last night. A few thugs breached Macy's, though they didn't seem to do much damage and most of them were caught. But panic is nearby and today's curfew is set for 8:00 p.m., three hours earlier than yesterday. Everyone knows the troublemakers are distinct from the protesters and use the large gatherings as cover for their mayhem. No one knows what will put an end to this craziness. Can curfews and police action deal with the bad guys while letting the good guys exercise their right to peacefully assemble and petition their government? Or will the criminal activity end only when the protests do? And when might that happen? As William Goldman famously said (of Hollywood), "No one knows anything."

As I write this, protesters are marching into Washington Square and the police have closed the public restrooms. So I need to go in order to preserve my right to go.

Now I'm in Hudson River Park where the restroom is still open. The sky is gray and hangs above Hoboken in layers of dark clouds. People exercise on the piers, walk their dogs, and stroll. But something is in the air and all we can do is wait and see. With the coronavirus we could help by staying home, wearing a mask, and keeping our distance from others. It never felt like enough, but it did "flatten the curve," as they say.

This new strain of infection—from civil unrest—seems beyond our control and the greater the police presence, the greater the chance of senseless violence. Instead of focusing on the small bands of looters, thousands of cops are surrounding peaceful protesters after curfew and executing a maneuver called "kettling," which none of us had ever heard of before and now everyone knows.

June 6

It's a beautiful Saturday and draws what seems like the biggest protests since the murder of George Floyd in Minneapolis. Thirteen days of marches and the crowds are getting bigger. I'm amazed they're still going and am impressed the protesters have mostly kept their cool, even when confronted with cops in riot gear and swinging batons. The looting has stopped, so perhaps the police are finally doing something right.

Washington Square is packed with people: protesters, bystanders, curious onlookers, and some, like me, who come to read the paper and catch some of the action. On the walk to the park, I notice restaurants doing a brisk business selling alcoholic drinks and serving as mini-social hubs for folks desperate for a bit of interaction. Most establishments still have plywood up, but find ingenious ways of opening parts of their storefronts to the sidewalk and their customers. In the park, there's a festive feeling—less angry and more optimistic than before. I see a few tables offering free water and snacks and watch people eager to participate in what seems like a historic movement. Something in the moment is calling all of us out of hibernation, if only to see what's going on.

June 7

De Blasio finally lifts the curfew today, and the city is scheduled to start "reopening" tomorrow. Cases and deaths are down significantly. The protests continue and opinion polls show a growing percent of the American public supporting the Black Lives Matter movement. The country as a whole seems finally to be recognizing the deeply rooted and sprawling nature of racism—how it affects everything from the daily interactions of Black people with the police to disparities in health, income, and opportunity between people of color and White America. The protests have touched people in a way that most others in the past have not. Perhaps it's timing, coming at a moment when most people are working from home and can take an hour or so to join in or at least watch.

Instead of enormous gatherings at major locations like the National Mall in DC or the Great Lawn in Central Park, the protests tend to be modest in size—a few hundred people here, a couple of thousand there—and they roam the city, occupying

Washington Square for forty-five minutes, then marching up University Avenue to Union Square. I've seen them at Sheridan Square, which is pretty darn small, and wandering down Seventh Avenue. The decentralized, fluid nature of the rallies makes them more accessible and perhaps less threatening. You don't have to go far to find one or make much of an effort to engage at least tangentially with one. That may explain why they are touching a lot of people and changing public opinion, even as their size is dwindling. They aren't big, but seem to be omnipresent—in more than 120 cities in the US and now abroad too.

Are we finally at a turning point? Or is this just another moment of false hope? New York has suffered greatly during the lockdown and will remain hobbled as long as Broadway theaters, museums,

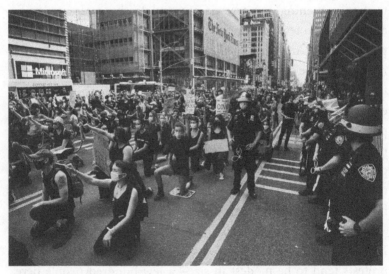

FIGURE 16
Police and Black Lives Matter demonstrators in midtown Manhattan. Photograph by Erica Lansner.

and other cultural institutions are closed or drastically limited in their operations. It will be many months before office buildings, stores, restaurants, and clubs are once again filled with people and probably years before the economy fully recovers. But if we become a more just and humane society as we stumble forward, all the pain we are currently experiencing may be worth it.

Protests, Riots, and Retirement

Richard Brea

In late May 2020, the killing of George Floyd by Minneapolis, Minnesota, police sparked demonstrations in New York City and throughout the United States. In June, the New York City Police Department disbanded anticrime units, arguing that they were an outmoded form of policing that alienated communities and too often were involved in shootings of civilians. Many police officers, however, believed they were an important tool for fighting crime. At the end of June 2020, Richard Brea retired from the New York City Police Department to work in the security industry.[14]

IT WAS A very challenging time for law enforcement not just here in New York City, but throughout the country. Officers were viciously attacked; precincts and police cars were set on fire. And yet, there was no support from our elected officials. I personally felt that the New York City mayor at the time was a coward; he used the NYPD as a scapegoat to protect his political ambitions. He was willing to say and do anything, just to appease the angry mob. But it didn't work. The mob got bigger and angrier, and his political ambitions failed miserably. But more importantly, I no longer wanted to be a pawn in this losing game.

Against his wishes, the officers of the 46th Precinct gave Brea a robust send off with bagpipes, a restored police car, and a helicopter fly by.

I love my cops. I love my community. I love this department. This department treated me very well.

At the time there was a part of me that didn't want to leave because I felt that I was leaving my cops behind. And I felt guilty about that. I certainly didn't want a sendoff. It wasn't the right time for it.

And someone close to me said, this sendoff is not for you. It's for them. It's for the cops. They feel like they've been beaten down so much. Everyone has abandoned the police. Every media commentary is negative, and the cops need something positive. Some of them felt, *finally*, someone, is speaking up for us.

It was very nice.

I miss the cops. I was fortunate to work for a good community. A lot of great people.

But very challenging times.

Broken Systems

Alexandra L. Naranjo

When she reflected on the pandemic, Alexandra L. Naranjo of Staten Island criticized the police (a sentiment not associated with her borough) but also noted, as did others in Staten Island, that Black Lives Matter protests there were not accompanied by the looting and violence seen at some protests in other boroughs.[15]

THE GEORGE FLOYD murder was a senseless, barbaric example of a corrupt justice system in this country. Sadly, he is only one on a long list of African Americans who have been unlawfully gunned down by the bullies in blue we call police. Though, at the same time, I think it was a horrible tragedy that became the catalyst we needed for reform, carried by the outrage of citizens. I am currently upset to see that it may have been short lived.

This particular case definitely impacted my view of Staten Island. At base, I always knew racism had its roots here. Mainly on our south shore. The severity of it I didn't really comprehend until I saw and heard statements on the subject with my own ears. People I grew up with, went to school with, not only making jokes about a man's death, but becoming more and more brazen with public threats. It really opened my eyes to the insidiousness of generational racism.

I did not participate in the protest. Largely due to work and scheduling conflicts. But also because I feared getting injured in the process, as I already have multiple physical injuries that keep me from being active a large part of the time. Honestly, I am still extremely disappointed in myself for letting fear get the better of me here. Because if taking a risk for something you believe in isn't worth it, then what is?

Like others interviewed by the Staten Island Coronavirus Chronicle project, she draws a contrast between protests on Staten Island and in other boroughs.

From what I remember, I believe the protests here weren't quite as agitated, or violent maybe is the word I'm looking for. I believe this is for two reasons. One, being it is a small island, and the repercussions for such things would be more concentrated. Less ways to leave or escape fallout in a bordered environment with notably less transportation options. Two, being that there are less degrees of separation here. Any violent situation has a higher likelihood of impacting someone you know, their brother, best friend, aunt, or your mother's dentist. It is harder to be anonymous here.

I think it is most important to understand the psychological and social impact this pandemic has had. I feel like the discussion, at the forefront, has been mostly financially/economically driven. About people losing work and some not being able to feed their families. I believe that this has been slowly addressed. Not well, but minimally addressed.

When it comes to the psychological, no one has moved a thumb to fix it. People at this point have experienced almost a year of isolation to varying degrees, which greatly affects the human psyche. Now, the powers that be are trying to usher those same people back into the roles they played prior without so much as a complimentary therapy session.

People have changed, and getting back to work will be the least of their acclimating issues. So much will go back into "getting back on track." Though this pandemic has unveiled all of the holes in citizen care that have been brushed under the rug for decades. Health care. Child care. Stagnant minimum wage despite higher production and profit. Wealth disparity. Weak policy making. Broken justice system. Environmental complications and the oil

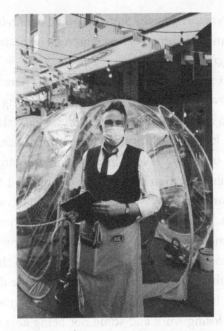

FIGURE 17
Masked waiter, Upper West Side of Manhattan, November 2020. Photograph by
Paul Margolis.

industry. Higher education. Housing. The list is quite literally endless in my eyes. Banking systems and Wall Street.

So many of our systems are broken, and this pandemic made so
many of them glaringly obvious. At this point, I'm really just waiting to see if any of it will change, or if people will miss "normal" so
badly that the entire country will stick its head back in the sand.

Opening Up

Kleber Vera (Flame)

Kleber Vera, an LGBT activist and resident of Jackson Heights in Queens, works as a hair stylist and performs in drag as Flame.[16]

I'M NOT SURE when the lockdowns started easing for everybody else, but I know for myself, I started easing my own personal restrictions when the protest started for George Floyd. I was very upset and outraged about that and I felt compelled to be out there marching on the streets for justice.

And I remember the very first protest I went to here in Jackson Heights. It was the first time in months that I was around so many people in one space. Even though everyone was masked, everyone was socially distant—as much as possible—it was just still very surreal to go from not seeing anybody (except for the grocery stores) to being in a crowded area. So that was very weird.

It was horrible situations and horrible circumstances that got me out there. It also made me realize that it is possible to be outdoors as long as you wear masks and remain distant to be safe.

So that kind of opened up a world of possibilities for me. Aside from marching to all the protests, I started going out on my own a little more, going to parks. I started riding the buses, I started exploring the neighborhood.

Exploring Queens

It was really incredible to think that I've been living in Queens for fifteen years, and there's so many parts of Queens that I haven't even seen just because I was usually so busy going to work, going home, going to work, going home. So that's actually a little nice, just exploring my area a little bit more.

I started seeking out other ways that I could help the community. I really miss doing hair. So I started doing hair at Travers Park in Jackson Heights either for free or by donations. Through posting pictures and videos of myself doing that someone reached out to me from NY1 and said they wanted to do a news story about that because I thought it was a really wonderful idea.

The public park became a space to meet people. It was just nice to see people out there trying to have some sense of normalcy.

As far as other public spaces like bars and nightlife, I was really into the Jackson Heights bar nightlife scene, especially the LGBT bar nightlife scene. I would go out pretty frequently. I went out once to go to a bar during the pandemic and it was just really strange having it be all outdoors. It kind of felt like Mardi Gras, like New Orleans.

I like that the bar scene has moved outdoors because obviously it's just safer, but I miss being in the music and the dark-lit ambiance of the bars. I didn't really enjoy it so much as an outdoor scene, especially now in the winter, which is why I only went once.

Activism

I discovered the food pantry out of necessity really. I couldn't afford to pay my bills, let alone buy food and feed myself. I heard of this LGBT food pantry called Love Wins Food Pantry. And I thought it was a wonderful idea. So I went there to get food— I think it was June-ish, around Pride—and I fell in love with the atmosphere. I started volunteering with them and I've been doing that since.

I noticed trans women of color being represented and other members of the LGBT community represented. And I thought it was so wonderful, not just that they were giving free food away (because that was my main reason for going) but something really resonated in me seeing that representation and I wanted to get involved.

Love Wins Food Pantry is LGBT run for LGBT people, but no one is turned away. So anybody can come receive free food. That is every Friday at 11:30 a.m. at Friend's Tavern, which is a local gay bar here in Jackson Heights. It's on the corner of Roosevelt Avenue and 78th Street.

This is LGBT run for LGBT people, but we do not discriminate. Straight, cis, everybody is welcome. So please come get free clothes. We don't limit the amount of clothes that you can get, and we don't judge. A lot of times we have families that are in need, but they also want to take some clothes to bring home or to send to their families, and you know, their countries of origin, that's fine as well.

I was so inspired by Love Wins Food Pantry, I wanted to have a clothing drive that had a similar LGBT representation. And me being a nonbinary person, I thought it'd be really fun to kind of do these weekly events in drag. I could be out there, showing LGBT representation and still being able to help the community.

I started Free Clothing Queens because the other organization where I was volunteering doing a free clothing drive closed down, and I love the idea of Love Wins Food Pantry with the LGBT representation. I wanted to combine the two.

With the help of a few other volunteers from Love Wins Food Pantry, I created this event and that's been wonderful going out once a week in full drag, giving out free clothing to the community, organizing events, helping people out. It's been very, very rewarding and it's been really nice to see it grow. We have like ten regular volunteers and a few other people that come once in a while to help.

We've done most of our events in Woodside, we've done events locally here in Jackson Heights, in Corona. Unfortunately, because of lack of transportation, we haven't been able to hit other neighborhoods, but I would like to go to Jamaica, the Rockaways, you know, other places that were also really hit by COVID. Especially in the wintertime, coats are really expensive. It's really nice for me to be able to go up to a family while in drag saying "here, here's some free clothing for you and your kids" and having them receive that and appreciate that.

Mutual Aid Online

Through ACQC, AIDS Center of Queens County, I started also doing these Facebook live events where I would talk to people about self-care and how we can all help each other. We also started doing Zoom meetups every Monday, and that's been really fun because it's helped keep the LGBT community together. So I've been keeping myself pretty busy.

It's been really good to get all the guys that were involved before COVID to get us all doing stuff together again, but it's also been nice to open it up to other people that could not have attended the event in person before. I have invited my LGBT friends from all over the world, Europe, Africa, from all over. And it's been really nice to welcome them into this Zoom space.

I've gone to Travers Park and gathered a group of friends together that have small kids and have done live readings to children in the park in drag. I think that's very important to continue doing that as well just to teach kids empathy and understanding and love and talk about, you know, anti-bullying and issues like that. So literally everything that I did pre-COVID, I started doing again on my own smaller scale, just not really been able to get paid for it. I just can't wait to get to the point where I can start doing it again for a living because the bills still keep coming.

And it's been really wonderful, just getting to meet my neighbors, being able to help them appreciate us as LGBT people.

Jackson Heights has always been a pretty LGBT friendly neighborhood, but there's still some homophobia, transphobia. It's nice to see them enjoying our help.

I think people see us in a different light now. Before they might've just have seen us as a nightlife people, people that walk the streets at night, going from one bar to the other, one club to the other. Now they see us in daylight helping out the community.

It's really mutual aid. We all help each other out. This is not a competition. It's not about, who's better at distributing and providing for the community. No, we're all in this together. We all want to help each other.

I went through a lot of depression in the beginning of this, and then once I started getting really busy with these side projects, these mutual aid projects, that's been really emotionally rewarding. But then when the winter hit, we have this new strain, that's been stressing people out, with the cold weather. I haven't been quite as active as I was before, and I haven't been leaving the house as much because of that. So I'm kind of back to the start dealing with depression, anxiety. I see there's no signs of things getting back to normal for me; financially, relationship wise, haven't really been able to see my family and friends, and it's still taking a toll. But I got through it the first time I'll get through it the second time. If there's a third and fourth time, I'll get through that as well. Just try to stay positive. But I would say definitely I've been very affected emotionally by this.

So I hope everybody gets through this well and happy and sane. I know that's what I'm trying to do.

"I'd Like to Think I'm an Optimist"

Patricia Tiu

Patricia Tiu, who worked as a nurse at New York–Presbyterian/ Weill Cornell Medical Center during the first surge in the spring of 2020, saw some improvements by late May.[17]

MY HAIR IS finally growing back, which I wasn't too worried about, I wasn't the only one who lost hair due to stress.

Toward the beginning of May is when we started seeing progress. We were able to clear out our OR [operating room] and our PACU [Post Anesthesia Care Unit] in the beginning of May. Unfortunately you had some patients that died. In terms of our equipment, my hospital has been a lot better. We are definitely given the gear that we need when requested but it is also still monitored. We are still being emailed or advised to conserve, which is definitely understandable. Our N95s are still kept in our manager's office, but when needed we are able to take them.

In terms of mental health I would love to tell all my nurses and essential workers and anyone who's struggling: please, please reach out to anybody, whether that's seeing a counselor, a friend, doing an activity. What we went through and what everybody is going through is not easy. I don't think I've had real time to actually process everything that goes on. I did start seeing the counselor.

For the most part I feel okay, but I do have my times where I'm very upset. I could have a beautiful day, the weather was amazing and everything was great and suddenly I'll be really upset. Or I could just be sitting here just like this and I'll just start crying. And I don't understand why. And I can be completely happy, I can even be with friends, and all of a sudden something just doesn't feel right. So for anyone who is struggling; please, I advise you please go speak to somebody, it will only help.

What we went through is not normal and what we're going through is not normal. There are a lot of other issues that COVID has brought out that we know of—job losses, people not being able to eat. I myself have been volunteering. I've been delivering food, I've been preparing food.

Different experiences

Everybody has a different experience. Someone who is stuck working from home has a different experience from me where I'm going in the hospital. Someone that is working in Elmhurst Hospital will have a different experience from someone that is working in like Long Island Jewish. There's so many different experiences, just know that together we could get through it by raising awareness and helping each other.

I still, from time to time, do check up on the patients that I have taken care of.

It brings so much joy to see that some of these patients are doing somewhat well, possibly off the ventilator. And then it breaks your heart to see the patients that are still on the ventilator. That have been on the ventilator for more than forty days and you just know the chances are just getting slimmer and slimmer. And then you have the ones that just didn't make it.

Typical day if I'm not working, usually go home, eat, maybe exercise or play basketball at open gym just with the community around here in Fresh Meadows or with my friends. Or go to the bar, have a drink or have dinner with friends or brunch. And then obviously play with my dogs. I have two dogs.

I ended up staying in Times Square Sheraton and I'm actually still there. For whatever reason, this hotel didn't have a microwave for the first month and a half. And we had no fridge, I have to ask for a fridge and thankfully they put a fridge in my room. But it was definitely a struggle being able to cook for yourself. I brought a blender, I brought a rice cooker. I don't eat out every day and I'm usually eating at home. So that was a struggle. What was nice is that they did have a shuttle that came back and forth.

Proud to be a nurse

The nurses that I work with every day, I'm extremely proud of them. Everyone stepped up, every single one of those nurses took initiative and didn't say no. It makes me so proud to be a nurse. Our nurses acted as not just registered nurses, they acted as doctors, they acted as respiratory therapists. They acted as the nursing assistants. They acted like the cleaning services. We emptied out our own garbage. We cleaned our own floors. Nurses and medical staff are really superheroes.

I'm genuinely proud of all the nurses that have stepped up during this time because it was not easy. They really did the impossible.

The clapping at seven really made me feel good. You may have a nurse who had such a crappy shift, patients might have died on their shift and as they're walking out, they hear somebody cheering. It makes a difference. It uplifts the spirit.

I miss seeing my friends and I miss playing basketball. It's just like little things like that.

You've just got to tell yourself it's going to come back one day, we just don't know when. God willing my family is safe and will stay safe.

Changes

Health care needs to change, at least American health care.

I'd like to think I'm an optimist. After the protests, I usually go with my coworkers and get a drink. It's been very refreshing to be able to sit down and have a conversation about the protests, about health care, about COVID. Just to have those conversations has been really good.

What else have I been doing for fun? Playing with my dogs is fun. [*laughs*] It doesn't take much for me to have a good time. I usually see light in something that makes me smile, even if it's the most minimal thing.

I ended up saving a lot of money during COVID. There was nowhere to go. No online shopping, no eating out, no dinners, no going to the bars or clubs or any of that stuff.

I'm constantly changing and growing for the better. I've definitely become more proactive in politics. I've always was proactive in public health but now actually using my platform to really try to educate everybody. I do believe I'm going to be a future leader. I don't think I'm going to be running for Congress but a leader—if there are young people out there that are looking into the nursing career or who need help with something, I feel like I'd be able to guide people. I've had people already talking to me about getting into nursing.

I am in school right now in Hunter College to get my psychiatric nurse practitioner degree. And a main reason I did that was because I wanted to kind of tackle the issues of domestic violence and human trafficking and woman's mental health, as well as public health in general, addressing disparities, helping immigrant families with health care because I feel like they're very underprivileged.

And with COVID and with this movement, it has only made me more knowledgeable of how our government reacts and treats the people.

I really didn't open my eyes till now and I think that having this knowledge and experience is only just going to make me a better leader. That's how I feel and hopefully it happens.

Discrepancies

Keerthan Thiyagarajah

Rich neighborhoods seemed to bounce back faster than working-class neighborhoods. Keerthan Thiyagarajah moved from his parents' home in Jackson Heights, Queens, to midtown Manhattan during the pandemic. Living with his girlfriend near the United Nations, he saw differences in how COVID-19 was experienced.[18]

MY PARENTS KNEW I was living with my girlfriend. They would drive over whenever they could, they would go to Costco, do their shopping and our shopping at the same time, and then they would drop it off in the city for us. And that was the only time we mingled face to face. But for the most part, everybody stayed home. I think that's the thing I struggled with the most, my family struggled with the most.

We're living in Midtown, two blocks away from the UN, a very wealthy upscale neighborhood. My girlfriend got a great price on an apartment, so why not? She was a college student at the time too, at Pace University. It was her final semester.

You can definitely see the discrepancy between the middle-class people in Jackson Heights to the wealthy upscale people working in Midtown. One of the big things I remember in Midtown was an imposed lockdown and curfew because of the rioting and the Black Lives Matter movement.

I was on East 50th Street and the precinct was one block away. And there was a barricade of police officers on Second Avenue, just blocking down the whole street, telling everybody to get home. And I remember them yanking off a delivery driver doing his job. He's delivering food to people and yanking him off the bike and beating him with a baton. And that was one of the biggest things I saw. I remember seeing it on the news. I'm like, that's literally up the block for me. That's like a hundred feet away from me that I watched that happen on the news.

And I got out, I left the apartment, I stuck my head out the window just to see like what the hell's going on outside. That was one of the craziest things I think I saw during that that time.

A lot more privilege in the city, in Manhattan. The city was getting a lot more people tested before anybody else. Restaurants were opening up way faster in the city.

When I went back home to Queens I would see everything still shut down, nobody was planning to do anything. There was no sign of people opening up stores or people going back out. But you can definitely see people in the city going out about daily lives. And I think the city opened up way, way sooner than any other borough.

I don't think the middle and lower class had the same resources available to the upper class. Upper-class people had a lot more opportunities and a lot more resources available to them. I think that was one of the big things that I witnessed during the pandemic.

After the Surge

Phil Suarez

Phil Suarez, a paramedic, saw a lull in the pandemic in the late spring and summer of 2020.[19]

IT WAS BEAUTIFUL. It was no traffic. [*laughs*] People still didn't want to go to the hospital. And there was no traffic. [*laughs*] It really was like nice in a sense. And I don't know if that's kind of mean or kind of selfish to say. But it was suddenly you had time to breathe, and you had time to process. It was crazy.

The drop-off in COVID-19 cases
Looking back, I felt that it came in very violent, and it left as abrupt. It was suddenly it was poof. It was gone it seems like. It wasn't gradual—it was steeper, like all of a sudden it started dwindling, which goes to show the stay in place worked. The social isolation worked. To us, to me, it felt like all of a sudden it was just gone. You were still getting it, but not that intensity that we had in those three weeks.

COVID-19 and racial disparities
I was surprised that people were surprised. "Oh my god. The colored people are doing worse." They always have. What's the shocker here?

They are targeted by the fast food industry. Their access to health care is not as good as many others. And they have higher comorbidities because of social issues. So that they would fare worse in a pandemic is kind of like—to me it was—like yeah. They always fare'worse. I was just shocked that even public health officials were taken back by it. Like what's the shocker here?

I guess what was surprising and what we still don't know now is why males were targeted, fare worse. Latino males and things like that. That was one of the things that was very intriguing that I definitely saw a trend. I definitely saw more males faring worse than women.

Heading into the winter

I survived the first round. I somehow walked away without getting it. I have no antibodies.

So I feel better. I have more knowledge. I don't feel as hopeless as I did in the first round.

COVID is a really bizarre beast. I had this woman that's eighty-nine years old. Tremendous amount of comorbidities. Obesity, high blood pressure, diabetes, the whole thing. And she was like three and a half weeks post COVID. She survived it. It's incredible.

It's dangerous. It's all luck, this thing.

I put my guard down through the summer. Mostly wearing surgical masks. I'm back to wearing N95 on every emergency. I'm taking more precautions. I always sanitize everything in the ambulance between patients. So definitely I've put up my guard for the perceived second wave.

Beyond that, just hunker down. I think that we all need to sacrifice 2020. If we sacrifice 2020 and just stay in place, enjoy your family, enjoy your surroundings, I think we would be in a better place in 2021.

Drawn-Out Deaths

Richard Jenkins (pseudonym)

Even as the first wave of the pandemic eased, Dr. Richard Jenkins (a pseudonym) noticed after-effects that lingered.[20]

THERE WERE A chunk of people who had come in with COVID in April and I feel so bad for them. Even though the COVID part of what brought them in had presumably resolved, they had all sorts of cascading injuries to other organs. It started with a really bad pneumonia but they ended up getting so many complications. They had such a degree of multiorgan failure that they were just permanently on dialysis.

A lot of them were not able to come off sedation. Or when they came off sedation, they weren't really waking up. And even though they weren't brain dead, they had developed enough neurological injury that it wasn't clear whether they'd ever return to their normal selves.

A lot of families didn't really want to accept that, particularly because they couldn't even be there to watch their course. They're thinking of every heroic movie where their family member wakes up. But realistically, we were just kind of keeping them alive with dialysis and machines until they eventually withered away and died.

So there were a lot of people who had these really drawn-out deaths, to put it in the most blunt way possible, over two months.

His understanding of COVID-19

I've definitely learned some things. When you watch a movie about a disaster, after a month or two the brilliant scientists have figured it all out and have solved the problem. And this is much, much slower than any of that.

The toll COVID-19 took on him
Emotionally, I've gotten a lot more anxious about things.

I had one episode where I was having a pretty mild argument about something not substantial with my wife. And I all of a sudden kind of had some flashbacks to when I would be with the charge nurse trying to decide among the fifteen people who didn't get dialysis who were supposed to, which three were going to get it. And for some reason I just started obsessively thinking about it. And I left the apartment and walked for like an hour. And just went onto a bench and cried for a long time.

I don't think I have PTSD because that was only one time. I don't think about it all the time. I'm able to function normally and all that. But something's changed. Something's changed. I definitely have a little bit of a darker color on things than I did before.

His biggest source of support
Definitely my wife. It's not even a question. We've been through this entire thing together. I've been there to support her. She's been there to support me. I couldn't have done any of this without her. And she's definitely my go-to for all kinds of support.

My mom has been great, too. I've been calling her every day and just kind of always checking with each other about how we're feeling.

Racial disparities in the pandemic
In my hospital in New York, just because of the location of the hospital, 90 percent of the people we treated were Black or Hispanic. Maybe 10 percent were White, or very rarely Asian.

I didn't feel like we were, at least intentionally, giving differential treatment based on someone's race during the COVID pandemic. The way it felt like to me was that our Black patient population, and Hispanic patient population, were already just very sick in general. If I had a Black patient come into the kidney clinic who didn't have diabetes and high blood pressure, I get surprised.

Those diseases, those chronic conditions run so rampant. And it's pretty evident to us that there's issues with medication access. There's issues with access to good food. There's insurance issues. I feel like we all try to do our best, but we kind of face an uphill battle.

For instance, you get a patient who doesn't have good insurance and they probably wind up needing dialysis in a few months. But if they could just get a medication that lowers the potassium in their blood, that they can take chronically, you might be able to stave it off for a little while. But the medication won't get covered, and you're fighting with the company. And nothing is getting done, and it doesn't get authorized. And then you're like, "I have no choice but to start dialysis."

Things like that build up and I think contribute heavily to the overall burden of chronic disease. When COVID comes in, a virus that really hunts down people with bad chronic diseases and affects them the most, then the virus is going to be that much worse.

I've always felt like our patient population was so riddled with diseases that were so hard to control. Where diet became such an issue because they couldn't afford better food or they were dealing with so many social issues, like family members in prison. They're dealing with legal things or issues with child care. So many problems that me trying to emphasize that they need to pick up this medication and eat better and exercise probably sounds like a joke to them. How are they going to actually be able to do those things?

But meanwhile, because they're unable to do those things, all their chronic conditions are just getting worse and worse and we're getting less control over them. And then boom, COVID comes in and hurts them so much more.

There's also sometimes an issue of trust. I sometimes have encountered patients who are Black—and I haven't seen this as much with my Hispanic patients—who are pretty blunt that they don't really trust me. Straight off the bat, they'll just say, "I feel like you've given me too many meds and that you're experimenting on me," or that "these medications are really making me sicker and I ought to stop them."

And that's a really hard battle to fight because I understand there's a lot of historical context behind feeling that way. But I'm trying to give the best care I can and follow the standards and the guidelines. And I just try to be very open and be like, "Let me explain exactly why you're taking each medication, and why we do this and what our thinking is behind it and the evidence. And it's your choice, ultimately. I can't force you to do anything. But this is why we're doing it." And I think maybe that gets through to some people. But I feel like the burden of chronic disease and the inability to control those is the bigger issue.

In sociological studies of disasters, the people with strong social ties and community bonds fared best.

The patients I've had who had a family at home, that had secure caregivers and stuff like that, were just generally doing better. Even if they were in their seventies and had a lot of medical problems, if they had a robust home health aide that was seeing them and family that was taking care of them, you can kind of tell.

You get these seventy-five-year-olds who have a health aide who just doesn't know what their meds are, doesn't know anything, and is just sitting there. And those people, you just watch them crash and burn and get COVID and not do well and end up in the hospital.

And then you find people who, like, their son is there and they can answer questions about their medication and they're involved. And they're just as sick. On paper it's the same thing—seventy years old, diabetes, hypertension, heart disease. But they're not ending up hospitalized.

Anticipating Vaccines

Jessica B. Martinez

Jessica B. Martinez is a global health expert with a background in virology and infectious diseases. By October 2020 she was hopeful that vaccines would change the course of the pandemic.[21]

THERE WERE A couple of times in April when I actually was scared. I remember having a couple of those moments where your heart kind of palpitates. And not scared for me but just thinking, like, the enormity of what's happening. And now I think it's even worse and people are so numb to it. And people are walking around, not here in New York, people still wear masks and stuff, but in the rest of the country. In all my years of imagining a pandemic, I just always assumed that people would have this feeling of self-preservation. And I am sort of shocked that that didn't quite pan out the way that I expected it would.

I'm quarantined. I am one of those people who does not go out unless I absolutely have to. I'm not necessarily wiping down every piece of mail, but if I order food, I either pop it in the microwave where I can, or I wipe down the containers. I wear a mask everywhere, not just for myself but obviously for everyone else—I hope that other people wear masks for me.

I think the worst thing that I could possibly ever imagine is being part of a transmission chain. Because at this point, knowing everything that we know, anybody who's out there being reckless, I don't want to be dramatic but they have blood on their hands that they either infected someone else or they helped to pass on an infection or enabled infection transmission. And from my perspective, that's my fear. I would never want to feel like I did anything that would, in any way, shape, or form, help transmit the virus.

I don't mind being home with my husband. I'm happy to be home, I'm not one of those people who doesn't like my spouse, so we have a lot of fun together. And so that's been very nice. I don't mind working remotely. I'm fine with that. And I don't need to go to restaurants. I have socially distanced get-togethers with a few friends that I know have also been equally cautious and we'll sit six feet apart from each other in a park.

I miss my friends a lot. I get to see a few of them. A lot of them are not in the city anymore. And I miss my family.

Vaccines

I'm feeling a lot better now that the FDA put out their guidelines, because I am a huge proponent of vaccines. Give me any vaccine possible, I'll take it. I think vaccines are a modern marvel. And I think that they have saved millions and millions of lives, enabled and empowered millions and millions of individuals, and I think that vaccines are fantastic. And I love seeing this push of these companies spending dollars and money and time and effort to make these vaccines, and some of them are very exciting.

I will stand in line when it is my turn to get one. And what I mean by that is that I think that there are high-risk individuals, first responders, physicians, hospital staff, people who are at high risk from the disease itself, elderly people who are immunocompromised, they should all get it first. Then you get into the other population stratified by risk.

Race, the pandemic, and the difficulty of enrolling African Americans in vaccine trials and treatment

That's just a broader challenge in general in medicine. Underrepresentation.

I went to med school. Doctors are human. My classmates were as blindly biased, racist as any cohort within the population. So yes, I think when you see these numbers coming out that say an African American baby is three times more likely to die—all things being equal and all other things being accounted for and corrected for—I mean that just tells you something, doesn't it?

The pandemic and her relationship to New York City

Oh, I love my city. I love my city. I know that there are some neighborhoods and certain places that are seeing a spike but I am so proud of how this city has pulled together, with helping neighbors who couldn't go out, doing everything they could to try to help businesses stay afloat. And now doing what they can to try to keep our numbers low.

I would not want to be anywhere else but here in a situation like this. And we didn't leave—we had no interest in leaving, we never even considered leaving. And yes, you see the occasional person walking down the street that makes you want to kind of throw something at them and yell at them to wear a mask, but for the most part, people here got it and it's probably because a lot more people here saw people die than most people in other states. People take it seriously here.

We know our neighbors quite well. I would say collectively our neighborhood was very good about checking in and making sure that the individuals within our neighborhood who didn't feel comfortable going out had what they needed or some of the elderly were well-protected and had also what they needed.

Her worries going forward

I worry about the people who are least among us right now. I worry about the people who are on a fixed income who don't have the ability to shop around for the food or the sundries that are safest. I worry about people who are living in the shadows. I mean, we all take for granted that we have the little guy from the deli who's going to deliver your food, but who's taking care of that person? And elderly, fixed-income people who are living in multigenerational homes where the kids are feeling generally pretty infallible, living right next to their grandparents. Even in New York where we have a pretty good social safety net, there are far too many people who are slipping through it.

Yes, this pandemic has really laid bare how unequal our society is. And even worse, how comfortable some people are with that. How okay they are with it.

I wish people would wear masks more. God, it makes my blood boil. When I see these people who are just so entitled, claiming that they don't want to wear a mask because it's so hard to breathe, I mean—try wearing a mask for sixteen hours in the ER.

Have Faith and Fight

Maribel Gonzalez Christianson

By November 2020 the worst days of the pandemic were a memory and the Bronx had resumed some of the functions and appearances of pre-COVID-19 life. Nevertheless, evolving public health regulations to track and limit the spread of COVID-19, rising expenses, declining revenues, and customers who did not want to abide by public health regulations made work difficult. Maribel Gonzalez Christianson, proprietor of The South of France, a Bronx restaurant, struggled on and kept faith with her neighbors and customers.[22]

We're still hanging in there, still grateful that some months have passed and we're still here. We're still not knowing if we're going to be here for one month to the next because the situation is still very precarious. Very delicate, very doubtful, and we're still fighting. We're doing the best to stay open, to keep staff employed. And it definitely is a struggle. The biggest problem is the whole up and down, up and down. Some days are good, some days are bad.

I've lost about ten catering jobs, which was equivalent to over $40,000 in lost revenue. And those things are very impactful. You still have all the ongoing expenses, all these operating costs, and they've increased because of the outdoor dining. To cover outdoor dining, my insurance has gone up almost $3,000 a year.

You have to make more trips, you're spending more on gas, you have to buy less because you have to keep everything fresh. When you buy in bulk you're able to save, but when you have to buy in smaller amounts in order to keep everything current and fresh, it's more costly and it's more cumbersome.

I used to buy once or twice a week, and now I have to do like three or four times a week in lesser amounts. If I know I'm going to have thirty customers as opposed to one hundred I can't buy for a hundred because I'll have wastage.

Municipal regulations brought expanded business opportunities and additional expenses.

At the beginning they said you can have outdoor seating, and you can have roadway seating, which is on the street; you can block off some area in front of your location. I went out and I bought what I thought were acceptable barricades and put signage on them. That was well over $2,000. Within two days an inspector came and said, "Now there are new rules, new guidelines and specifications to follow, and these are not acceptable." To fulfill that and to have outdoor seating cost an additional unexpected $4,800 to get twelve barricades.

I understand having empathy for the city, this is all our first go around. And they're doing the best they can to help us and stay in business. They're flying by the seat of their pants. However, for a small business, when you're told one thing and then a couple of days or a week later, that changes, that's another investment. That's a big problem for us. We need clear direction.

I'm calling 311. I'm calling the mayor's office, the governor's office. I'm calling Small Business Affairs, I'm calling Consumer Affairs. I'm all over the place, trying to find out the latest guidelines. They set up this New York restart hotline for small businesses. And often, they didn't even know themselves. They said, "I'm sorry, we don't have the latest update information to give you on that yet." I often ask questions that they could not answer, and so that was extremely frustrating.

Moving forward, there has to be more concise and specific guidelines that we can all get in a timely basis and depend on and have assurance that we're not going to have an additional cost after that because there's going to be yet another change.

Aside from all the stresses of managing the operation on a daily basis, making sure that food is coming out on a timely basis, you also now have to be vigilant.

I'm constantly having to justify, explain, reiterate, repeat what the rules are.

"I'm so sorry you have to wear your mask."

"If you're sitting outside, you're welcome to use the restroom, but you have to put on the mask."

"You cannot hang out outside and stand holding a beer or an alcoholic beverage in your hand on the sidewalk talking, you can only consume when you're sitting down at the table. "

You're always being as polite as possible. There's so many rules to follow. People forget, they don't do it intentionally.

People are starving for socialization. I'm very much known as a cheers place, where everyone knows your name. Everyone is happy to see each other, and their inclination is to say hi and go up to them. But they forgot to put on the mask. And you're constantly having to play vigilance with all those details. And people sometimes get annoyed and I have had to turn away business with people that are not believers in using masks.

People get frustrated. They become defiant—"Oh, it's only for a minute" and "I'm only going to stand up for two seconds."

And you can't bend the rules. I didn't make them, I just have to follow them.

Now there are many more inspectors throughout the city in the five boroughs. And they're very vigilant, rightly so, and they come in unannounced, to spot check your place if you're not enforcing the rules. You're also required to keep a log of not only your employees' daily temperature, but of anyone that comes in to dine. At least one person per party has to provide the contact information in case of any illness.

And so they don't want to follow the rules. I can't risk what could very well be a $10,000 fine. So I've had to say no to customers and excuse them from the premises.

I am counting on my community to say that they are not only with us, but with all small businesses in all times. I think it's important that people realize that the mom and pops is America. And we hope that people realize that by supporting local small business, supporting your neighborhood, it's always worth it. And we strive to be worthy of that.

I remain positive that we'll be able to overcome this. I'm hoping that things will turn around for the better.

I believe in New York, I especially love and believe in my Bronxites. This cannot last forever. We will overcome, they will find a vaccine. We will end this. It's all incumbent upon us to take care of

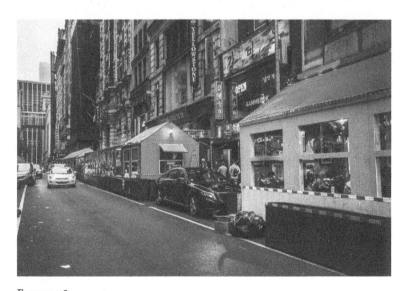

Figure 18
July 13, 2021: Dining sheds, Koreatown, West 32 Street, Manhattan. Photograph by Tom Pich, Corona Chronicles Collection, City Lore Archive.

our fellow citizens, our fellow Bronxites. We can't despair and we have to have faith and hang out a little longer.

We've overcome so many other things as New Yorkers, and we're strong and we're warriors. And so you have to have faith and you have to fight.

The Best Place to Be

Jessica B. Martinez

New Yorkers waited anxiously for four days to learn the results of the hotly contested 2020 presidential election, but when Joe Biden's victory over Donald Trump was announced on the morning of Saturday, November 7, the city erupted in celebrations. New Yorkers, recovering their talent for public festivity, gathered in parks and intersections, formed motorcades, and cheered from apartment windows. One of the celebrants was Jessica B. Martinez, a global health expert who had watched the progress of the pandemic with concern and fascination.[23]

I STAYED UP until about four o'clock in the morning on election night, that's when Michigan flipped over, and it was looking like

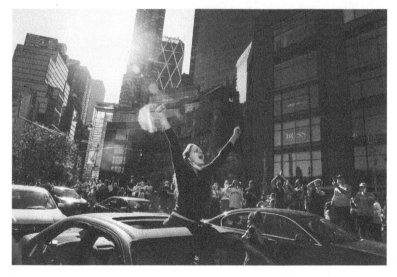

FIGURE 19
Columbus Circle, November 7, 2020: Exultation at a motorcade to celebrate Joe Biden's victory in the 2020 presidential election. Photograph by Erica Lansner.

Georgia was, and Arizona as well, and at that point I felt I could go to sleep. And Pennsylvania was trending in that direction as well. At that point, I actually felt optimistic. I won't say that I was certain but I was pretty sure that Biden was going to win, it was just a matter of time. We just had to be patient.

And then when he was declared the winner, being in New York City was just about the best place you could possibly be. People were running out in the streets with champagne. We did the same. Everybody was screaming, banging on pots. We did drive down through Times Square that evening, in sort of that promenade of cars that was going down and everybody was screaming and hollering. I mean it was fantastic. It was absolutely fantastic.

7

Vaccines and After, 2021

Americans like tragedies with happy endings, as novelist William Dean Howells once observed, and New Yorkers during the pandemic were no different.[1] Through long days of lockdowns, fear of a debilitating illness, and mounting death tolls, they longed for an end of their woes. Most of all, they pegged their hopes to the arrival of vaccines that would protect them from the virus that had robbed them of normal life. The vaccines, a triumph of science, arrived in December 2020. New Yorkers hoped that in 2021 they would break the back of the pandemic. But COVID-19 was not entirely overcome. It dragged on, vastly less deadly than it had been in 2020 but still casting a shadow over the city. Even with vaccines, more surges—driven by the Delta variant in 2021 and the Omicron variant in 2022—lay in the future. When they arrived, their presence mocked the highest hopes for the vaccines, even though shots did reduce your likelihood of getting infected and reduced the severity of infections.

The spirit of solidarity that marked the spring of 2020 endured, but it was marred by notes of division and denial that had been in the background since the earliest days of COVID-19. Some of this echoed the political divisions in the nation as a whole, but the city harbored its own hostilities that were illuminated or accelerated by the pandemic.

The first COVID-19 vaccine was administered on December 14, 2020, to Sandra Lindsay, a Jamaican-born citizen of the United States who was educated at the City University of New York and director of critical care nursing at Long Island Jewish Medical Center in Queens.[2] But widespread hopes of a quick and decisive rollout of the vaccine were dashed.

In New York City, a computerized system for making an appointment to get a vaccine was glitchy and inefficient.[3] Websites for registration were difficult to navigate even for experienced computer users. People eager to get their shot were sent to vaccine facilities far from their homes, and suburbanites were directed to facilities in the city where the need for vaccines for local residents was pressing. Worst of all, the internet-based system marginalized the very New Yorkers who were most in need of vaccines: old people and poor people with little access to the internet.

New Yorkers met the inefficiencies of the registration with resolution and ingenuity. They created apps and websites to help people beat the system, telephoned each other to let them know when appointments were becoming available at specific locations, and even volunteered to make appointments for people who needed help with computers. Gradually, the system responded. By the middle of April, at the peak of the vaccination effort, close to 100,000 doses of the vaccine were being administered daily. Cases, hospitalizations and deaths plummeted by summer.

Yet New Yorkers could never summon up a collective celebration anything like the joyful crowds that filled Times Square at the end of World War II. On July 7, 2021, the city mounted a ticker tape parade for essential workers. Spectators in the Canyon of Heroes on lower Broadway cheered nurses, doctors, first responders, health care professionals and other frontline workers. But reporters noted that the crowds were smaller than at other parades, in part because many downtown stores were still closed and because several municipal unions didn't participate because they were in contract disputes with the city.[4]

Indeed, the celebration was premature. For all the high hopes that surrounded the July 2021 ticker tape parade, there was another surge of COVID-19 yet to come. Equally troubling, the relief at being safer (but not permanently immune) from the virus was accompanied by debates over masking, vaccine mandates, school reopenings, and even the safety of the vaccines themselves.

Skepticism about vaccines was brewing for years before COVID-19 hit, drawing on everything from religious beliefs to a hostility to scientific expertise in general. By 2020, in a development that could make vaccine debates confounding, some antivaccine sentiment was drawing on ideas associated with Democrats and leftists: environmentalism (with its wariness on what we put in our bodies), feminism (my body my choice), and hostility to corporations (why trust Big Pharma?) Antivaccine sentiment was even more powerfully nourished by a libertarian strain in American conservative thought, a hostility to government-sponsored projects that had become central to the ideology of the Republican Party since the 1980s, and conspiratorial thinking among White nationalists and other Trump supporters about deep state plots in the federal government to subjugate true Americans.[5]

New York City was not a hotbed of antivaccine sentiment, but antivaxxers were a presence online and in demonstrations at Manhattan's Civic Center.[6] The slowness of some New Yorkers to get vaccinated—owing more to skepticism about vaccines than outright hostility—was rooted in the distrust bred in unequal access to medical care that has harmed poor people and people of color.

For some African Americans, a long history of unequal medical care, and a long memory of unjust treatment at the hands of medical researchers—who withheld syphilis treatments in the Tuskegee Experiment and studied Henrietta Lacks' cells without asking her permission—created a deep distrust of American medicine. (Nevertheless, in the pandemic they eventually overcame that distrust. By 2022 in New York State, the Kaiser Foundation reported, Blacks had been vaccinated at the same rate as Whites [71 percent], while 84 percent of Hispanics and 99 percent of Asians had been vaccinated.)[7]

This mistrust occurred against the background of a frayed safety net that left New Yorkers with uneven access to medical care. The recovery from the fiscal crisis of the 1970s had produced a city with significant social and economic inequalities. During the same period, a conservative ascendancy in national politics had attacked and undermined the universal social welfare programs of the New Deal and Great Society. New York in 2020 remained a socially liberal city, but the urban social democracy that had characterized it since the Depression was a diminishing presence. New Yorkers with low incomes, and people of color, fell through the holes in the city's safety net and had little access to doctors or caregivers they could trust. The city's institutional public health apparatus was strong, but its emphasis on chronic diseases—the lung cancer caused by smoking, the diabetes caused by sugary drinks—could make public health seem like a hectoring enterprise that criticized people for making bad lifestyle choices. All these trends undermined the idea of public health as a common good, grounded in a shared responsibility to protect each other. Instead, for many New Yorkers, health was a matter of personal choice and individual behavior.

Although more than 84 percent of New York City adults were vaccinated by November 2021, there was still resistance to the shots—especially among municipal workers. At the Department of Corrections, the vaccination rate was 51 percent; in the Police Department 70 percent; and in the Fire Department and Sanitation Department about 60 percent. Mayor de Blasio issued a mandate requiring city workers to get vaccinated to keep their jobs and offered $500 bonuses as an incentive. Legal challenges and demonstrations followed. In the end, 96 percent of municipal workers were vaccinated. But the slowness of the vaccine process, and the resentment sparked in some quarters, revealed a city at odds with itself. (Transit workers, whose work for the Metropolitan Transit Authority makes them state employees not covered by the municipal vaccination mandate, were reluctant to be get vaccinated: by November 2021 some 68 percent had received a shot.)[8]

Especially troubling were signs that New Yorkers were not only at odds over the vaccine, but hostile and even predatory toward one another. Scapegoating immigrants during epidemics has a long history in New York City, beginning in the nineteenth century with the false claim that it was the moral turpitude of Irish immigrants (and not dirty drinking water) that caused cholera. During COVID-19, some New Yorkers blamed Asian Americans for the pandemic. Verbal abuse, physical assaults, and even killings (which were difficult to designate as hate crimes because of legal definitions) left Asian New Yorkers feeling like a community under siege. Violence against Jews also surged to high levels, driven by a broader rise in White nationalism and anti-Semitism. At the same time, Jews clashed with each other over the value of masking.[9]

Ethnic tensions were accompanied by a rise in crime during the pandemic. New York City entered COVID-19 with historically low levels of crime, and the percentage increases that stoked headlines made things look worse than they were. Nevertheless, there was an undeniable rise in the level of fear in the city. Notorious but statistically unrepresentative crimes frightened subway riders. Shootings in which New Yorkers wounded or killed each other with firearms were a bigger and more revealing problem: from 2019 to 2020, the number of shooting victims in New York City, killed and wounded, jumped from 923 to 1,868.[10]

In 2021, the city experienced a political sea change. Governor Cuomo, who had already lost political support over his handling of COVID-19 deaths in nursing homes, was hit with multiple allegations of sexual harassment. His political standing collapsed. He resigned as governor in August 2021 and was replaced by Lieutenant Governor Kathy Hochul. In November 2021, Brooklyn Borough president Eric Adams, an African American and a former police officer who simultaneously critiqued police violence and vowed to make the city safer, won the mayoral election. The Black Lives Matter protests of only a year earlier were followed not by a turn to the left, but a more moderate course.[11]

With vaccines, New York left behind the darkest days of the pandemic. But the full impact of COVID-19 on the city was yet to be measured. The city's population fell from 8,804,000 in 2020 to 8,335,000 in 2022, and its economic recovery—so heavily dependent on office workers and service workers—was slower than in other places. In 2023, there were still many empty storefronts on city streets, real doubts over whether the city's office-based economy would ever return, and a painful shortage of affordable housing.[12]

If New Yorkers were "done with COVID," as a saying of the time went, COVID-19 was not done with them. Federal authorities declared the COVID-19 public health emergency to be over in May 2023. COVID-19 continues to evolve, however, and its future is uncertain.

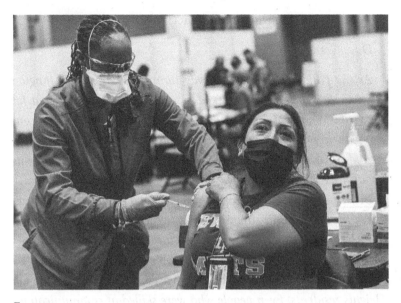

FIGURE 20
Jacob K. Javits Center, Manhattan, January 13, 2021: Maria Diaz, a transit worker, is vaccinated early in the vaccine campaign. Photograph by Marc A. Hermann, MTA/New York City Transit.

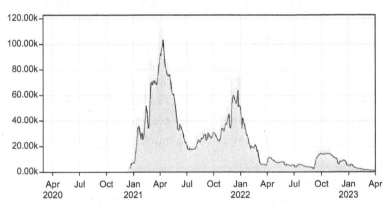

FIGURE 21
Daily and rolling averages of COVID-19 vaccine doses administered, April 2020 to April 2023. Chart: BetaNYC. Data: New York City Department of Health and Mental Hygiene.

Registration Nightmares and Vaccine Skepticism

Dave Crenshaw

As the pandemic burned its way through 2020, in Washington Heights, Dave Crenshaw worked to get people fed and tested for the virus. When vaccines finally came to his neighborhood, he confronted two problems: the logistical nightmare of getting people registered for their shot and the skepticism of some uptown residents about the value of vaccines.

In January 2021, NewYork–Presbyterian Hospital's vaccination site at the Fort Washington Armory between 168th and 169th streets quickly attracted people from across the metropolitan area. News coverage raised the issue of White people descending on a largely Black and Latino neighborhood to get vaccines ahead of Washington Heights residents. Even people who were skilled at communications technology had trouble making appointments with the complicated system, which required registration by phone or through websites that frequently broke down. For Washington Heights residents who spoke only Spanish or lacked access to computers or cell phones, it was almost impossible.[13]

PEOPLE WERE COMING from all over the East Coast to get vaccines at the Armory. We had to make a big huff about it, a big complaint about it, because our people couldn't even get appointments. What it took just to get registered was too much for the average person.

Crenshaw's Team Dreamers had been running track at the Armory for more than twenty-five years, and he knew people from both the Armory and NewYork-Presbyterian. He also had his enduring contacts across Washington Heights, such as Professor Robert Fullilove of the Mailman School of Public Health at Columbia University and

Maria Luna, a long-time Dominican American public servant in northern Manhattan.

I had a public health network. I had people I trust. I got my own professor, Robert Fullilove, and he got a family of professors. And between Mailman School of Public Health and Hunter College High School, I was getting the best information in the world, from people I trusted and love. We've known each other for decades.

I started working with Maria Luna. And Maria Luna was working with ARC, which has three centers for senior citizens in upper Manhattan, and the Northern Manhattan Improvement Corporation. And they were all working with NewYork-Presbyterian to streamline the system to get people appointments over the telephone.

Eventually Mailman had volunteers in the Armory. The Armory had the best site in the city because it was right here with Columbia. Nobody had better volunteers. Every ten feet they were asking, "Are you okay?" Once you got there, you were all right.

Late in July 2021, with the pace of vaccinations declining, the Mayor Bill De Blasio announced that the city would give $100 to anyone who received their first vaccination at a city-run vaccination site.

The $100 was huge. The $100 really did work. It really did change things.

You have to force people to take care of themselves. This is part of life. This gives you the extra energy and mojo. People were lining up.

But the biggest problem was you also had to show them how to get the $100. So the Black Health interns and the Mailman interns and the Dreamers would work a site. Somebody is going to help you get registered for the vaccine, someone's gonna help you fill out the paperwork you got to fill out. Once you get the vaccine, we're also going to show you how to get your $100. Our vaccine sites became like a community hub.

In Washington Heights, with a large Latino community and many Dominicans, Crenshaw worked with Spanish-speaking interns who could communicate with local residents, especially the elderly.

People didn't know who they could trust. So we became the place you could come and ask us questions.

With the training that Black Health and Mailman gave me I was able to speak facts, I was able to have good conversations. That number-one thing I learned as a coach is you don't tell somebody they're wrong. There is more than one truth. That's the simple fact. Your experiences in your life are going to determine your truth.

Crenshaw confronted the arguments of people who were skeptical about the value of vaccination and even thought it might kill them.

The biggest argument they would give is, "But what about if people are dying?"

So, who? Who do you know that died from the vaccine?

I can tell you fifteen people off the top of my head who I know that died from COVID. But you can't even tell me one. If that was really happening, you'll be able to name somebody you lost to the vaccine.

"Well, you vaccinate a lot of people, but dead people can't talk."

So let me explain something to you. I'm in my neighborhood. I'm doing my events in my area. If somebody dies from the vaccine, I'm the first one they're coming after, because I'm easy to find. I'm right here. I'm trying to make this work.

But here was the worst one to me.

"You do know they created the vaccine to kill you. You understand they're getting you vaccinated so you get killed."

But that theory, you lose with that one.

People were dropping every day in the beginning. The death rate was way higher before the vaccine came out. The vaccine was not speeding up death. It definitely slowed it down.

Folks were talking about chips so they could track you and follow you.

Yeah, but if you don't want to get tracked, you don't take the vaccine, you got to get rid of your phone also. You got a phone—they tracking you, baby.

But my thing was, where you getting your logic from? How long do you know them? Have you ever met him? Why you trust him?

My guy, Robert Fullilove, I know him. I know his ex-wife. I know the students he teaches, I know professors he works with, I know projects he was working on when he was in HIV and AIDS. I've trusted my life with him before this. He's not someone I met during the pandemic.

And one of the lines was, "This is something that White folks is using to kill Black folks, like they did in Tuskegee."

I'm like, you're not really looking at this because the White folks are trying to take all our appointments. They're lining up for this, that should tell you something right there.

It'd be one thing if they were just giving out the vaccine in the Black and Hispanic neighborhoods. But the vaccine was being distributed everywhere. People were going wherever they could to get vaccinated. And at every site you had people of color distributing it.

One Friday, Crenshaw was alerted that vaccines would be available the next day in Harlem, the neighborhood just south of Washington Heights. He went door to door in his building and took older people who needed shots to Harlem, where a worker asked Crenshaw if he had received a shot.

I said I ain't no senior. She comes back with a paper and says, "You're getting vaccinated today. Because we can't have people like you getting sick and not helping other people."

When she gave me the vaccine it was like she baptized me to get other people the vaccine. Because I know how I felt getting it. Now I could fight even harder. Now I could go even more.

The Second Shot: *New York, February 2021*

Rachel Hadas

New York City's computerized system for COVID-19 vaccination reservations was difficult to navigate and often matched vaccine recipients with vaccine centers far from their homes, as when the poet and Rutgers–Newark professor Rachel Hadas was sent from the Upper West Side of Manhattan to Canarsie, Brooklyn, for her second shot in February 2021. Getting vaccinated meant making a trip, meeting strangers, and seeing new sights after months of isolation.[14]

Vaccination lured us out of doors.
Approaching spring and the full moon
may also have helped draw everyone together.
But not too close. Not yet.
Through the cold courtyard, all around the block,
wound a line.
The wheelchair-bound, the leaners on their walkers,
these had priority—unwritten rule.
People were patient, even a bit cheery;
a spritz of subdued small talk.
One was no longer afraid, after a year,
to turn their masked face toward a stranger's face.
We couldn't wholly see each other;
we all could see the sky.
As you and I drove back from Canarsie—
the water out of sight but palpable
in the tremble and lambency of afternoon—
our hungry eyes were suddenly satiated
with a luxuriance of primary colors:
blood-red truck, yolk-yellow warehouse wall,
and two immensities, two shades of blue:
dark flowing river, overarching sky.

A Question of Trade-offs

Alexandra L. Naranjo

The vaccine rollout raised concerns for many New Yorkers. Alexandra L. Naranjo of Staten Island got her shot, but her questions endured.[15]

I'M A TWENTY-SEVEN-YEAR-OLD female, a college graduate, and identify with two separate ethnic cultures, being born both Puerto Rican and Italian. I'm currently working on additional schooling for political science and photography. I also identify as a recovering alcoholic, and for the last few years, have worked in the substance abuse and mental health treatment sector of the health care industry.

The COVID-19 pandemic definitely impacted my life. Not only on a day-to-day basis—transportation, difficulty getting hands on various products, an inability to take part in activities or hobbies one is used to, and the like—but also on a deeper level. My comfortability with interpersonal communication has been impacted in the long run. My community was impacted as well, but most specifically the community of recovering addicts I'm connected to. As someone who works in the field as well, we saw almost a 33 percent rise in relapses and deaths. It was an extremely hard year on this front in particular. Staten Island I feel (as to be honest I don't know the exact data) may have been impacted even more than the other boroughs due to a pervasive, conservative mindset that left people at risk. For example, "antimask" rhetoric.

I remember hearing about the vaccine being released in New York a few months ago but couldn't give you a timeline if I tried. Especially with the gradual rollout. My first thoughts were that

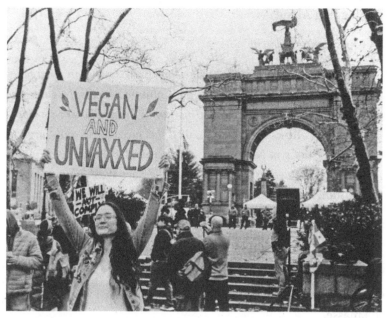

FIGURE 22
Antivaccine demonstration near Grand Army Plaza, Brooklyn, October 2021. Photograph by Paul Margolis.

there would be complications, and second, questioning whether or not the adverse effects (we know nothing about long term effects) would be worth the risks.

There are trade-offs for everything. But it is a bit more difficult to accept not knowing what the trade-off will actually be. At this point, I am fully vaccinated but still have anxiety about what this could mean for my future. Especially as a woman given that there are some issues concerning the impact it could have on conceiving a child.

Overall, though, I guess every vaccine had to start being administered to humans at one point.

Slogging Along

Christopher Tedeschi

During the summer of 2020 Christopher Tedeschi, an emergency physician and faculty member at the Columbia Medical Center and the Allen Hospital, moved with his family from Harlem to Upper Nyack, New York. In January 2021, he faced a second surge in COVID-19 cases in New York City; he was deeply involved in vaccinating people against COVID-19 at the Fort Washington Armory in Washington Heights.[16]

WE HAD THIS nice lull, and most of that time we spent making plans for what we anticipated for the fall. And then we started becoming busy with COVID again. The surge is at its height right now and we've been vaccinating people for the last week and a half, en masse.

We are busy. We are stretched, but we are nowhere near where we were in March and April. Since maybe November, we've been dealing with this simmering pot, but the pot has not boiled over. And if this week and the next ten to fourteen days are the peak, the way we anticipate, hopefully the pot won't boil over.

From a going to work point of view, we can handle this. We spent the summer making this plan, we know what our next step is; it's busy, there's sick people, but it's not overwhelming.

March was overwhelming. Now it's just a matter of fatigue. We've been doing this for a long time now and going through those motions every single day. The morale among a lot of our staff is a little bit low, despite the vaccine. We're slogging along far more than we are freaking out.

Our memories of this from eight months ago are people rolling in one after the other in extremis, and we're not seeing that now.

We're not seeing people come in the door who are about to die. We're seeing people who are sick. We're seeing people who need to be admitted to the hospital, maybe they get even sicker a few days later. But there isn't this sense of emergency that we had been seeing before. It is night and day in terms of what you see and hear and smell when you walk into the emergency department where I work.

Changes in the social fabric of his department
It's far more isolated. People are on guard more. The opportunity for social interaction has gone down so much. I don't really teach in person. I don't go to have my lunch in the conference room.

It's hard to even walk down the hall. You don't even recognize people a lot of the time. Sometimes you pass someone in the hallway, and they say, "Hey how's it going?" And I'm sure it's somebody I know well, but they're so wrapped up in PPE [Personal Protective Equipment] that you're really not so sure. So you have to look at their ID badge, and then by that time, you've walked by them. So there's definitely this distance that persists. And I think at least at work, it'll probably persist for a while.

Vaccines
We're vaccinating people wholesale now. I was vaccinated on December fifteenth, some time ago now. And it's a very profound experience. It's a huge change in perspective, certainly at work. I still wear all the crap that I've always worn. But there's a degree of, "I got my vaccine, I should be okay."

Now that we're vaccinating people in this huge space, it's really interesting to interact with people. It's actually very hopeful, and I'm usually pretty cynical about these things. There are people who have waited and waited and waited and drove six hours taking selfies after they get their shot, which is very different from the ER, where everyone is either appropriately or inappropriately miserable or mean and unhappy.

We're vaccinating more than two thousand people a day now. Maybe twenty-three, twenty-four hundred. And so you really can look around at the end of the day and say, "A couple of these people won't get critically ill because of this today. A couple of these people just won't die."

Vaccines and skepticism

We're having a real problem at work getting certain groups of people to get vaccinated. And I'm not surprised. Because the hospital's a huge employer, there's thousands and thousands of people in that group. But the way it was targeted was, to my mind, probably not that effective.

There's a really big diversity of people where I work. A huge proportion of our staff are primarily Spanish speaking, or Spanish is their first language, who work in service industry type jobs. And if you look at the sort of material that the hospital produced—"The vaccine is coming"—it's geared to people who really have a degree of facility with being online and understanding science, and that stuff just doesn't resonate with most of the people that are refusing or hesitant to get vaccinated now.

Our security guards are a particularly hesitant group. They were all there with us. They saw the trailers. They know what happened. Watching a six-minute video from the COO [Chief Operating Officer] of the hospital, who's a surgeon, probably doesn't fly that well with a lot of our staff. I don't watch it. I can't imagine they're going to watch it. I delete it, you know.

To get an appointment at our vaccination site, you have to log onto the app and register, and have a pretty aggressive degree of computer savvy. Especially at the beginning, the population lining up to get vaccinated was clearly a very self-selective kind of savvy population.

And there was a reaction to that, and now the people that were in charge of this are reserving several hundred appointments a day for our local population, and reaching out in English, reaching out in Spanish. But it's a real challenge.

It's very labor intensive. If you're sixty-five years old and a patient of our clinic system, there is this group of people now that are working to reach out and say, "Hey, we can make you an appointment." I think they've just implemented a text message system where the patient will get a text, and if they just click a link in the text, then they can reserve their spot, which is way simpler than the other kind of procedure.

And there's still hesitancy on top of that. That doesn't address the hesitancy, it just addresses the access.

Getting vaccinated

Believe it or not, even in the vaccination center, I've seen one or two people get in line and get out of line, and get in line, and get out of line.

I've had many, many conversations with our staff—some of the security officers, several nurses. Many of those people are either Latinx, or primarily Spanish speaking, or Black. We have a lot of West Indians that work with us. And a lot of them I have known for years. I had a conversation the other day with a security officer who is a Latino guy who I've known probably for ten years.

And I feel they trust the doctors, they kind of trust people they know, and you're able to have a frank conversation. And this particular person said, "You know, I don't know, I'm just waiting for them to work the kinks out of it."

To which I said, "What do you mean work the kinks out?"

"Well you know, we work with this guy who got the vaccine, and like later that day, he had a 102 fever, and he's been in bed for a week, and he's got a cough."

And clearly, the person he's describing probably had COVID, not anything to do with the vaccine. But as soon as that connection is made and your buddy is in that position, you stop and think.

I had another conversation with a security officer who is I think West African, who had clearly read a lot of stuff online, a lot of false technical information. And who said, "I was here this whole time, and I didn't get it yet."

And those are conversations that can go on for a long time. I've definitely talked to one or two people that came back to me a week later and said, "Hey I got my shot." And so there's a little bit of early adopter fear there. But I don't think it's helpful to say, "Here is why you should get the shot. And because it works, and the data shows this."

Taking a little bit of a time to try to meet that person where they are is helpful. Although it takes a lot of unpacking. "Well, I want to wait and work the kinks, see if they get the kinks worked out" is actually kind of a conversation you can start having, because you can say "Well, they tested it on these people, and we know the side effect."

But when someone says, "I think it's some kind of conspiracy about something," that's actually a lot harder. As time goes on, hopefully people will see people they know and trust do it, because watching the video online from the COO of the hospital is not doing anything.

Reflections on how he has changed since his interview in July 2020

I feel older. I'm approaching my fiftieth birthday. A lot of things just make me feel older, and hopefully that will change. I'm very lucky to be in good physical shape.

I'm also a lot more grateful for a lot of things. I've seen a lot of people get sick and lose jobs, a lot of hardship. I'm grateful for a lot of the things that my family is lucky enough to still have. And I mean that sincerely.

Social skills atrophied

Things are going to be different for a long time. Whether it's just the way we work, where I work, or the way we interact.

It's been kind of isolating to be honest with you. I certainly feel my close relationships with my friends have suffered.

To have a frank conversation with a friend even requires some attention. I just need a minute of quiet, rather than engaging another human being. But that's a self-fulfilling prophecy. Once you get out of the habit of exercising that muscle, then you don't exercise that muscle.

The start of the Biden administration makes him optimistic.

It's clearly, to my mind, politically an improvement. The very specific things that will need to get done will not happen overnight. It's like changing the course of a cruise ship, you have to make this big turn. But I clearly believe that the leadership that will be in place will have a real world effect on the way things happen.

We're seeing it now with vaccines. You can only hope that the policy decisions that get made have a real trickle down effect. I think it will.

In terms of information, I'm optimistic that that'll make a real difference. Not just because there'll be more positive messages, but because there'll be fewer negative messages. And just getting rid of the negative messages I can only hope will go a long way. Maybe that's naïve.

Dealing with trauma

It's smart to frame this all as a trauma, a really drawn-out, protracted, slow-burning trauma. I'm not sure we've all come to process it as much as might be helpful. There are plenty of resources out there, but just collectively processing it, probably has a good way to go. And not just in terms of the illness, but just the social distancing and the social isolation and the kids and all of that stuff will take some processing.

Changes and Challenges

Jessica B. Martinez

By early March 2021, life in the Hamilton Heights section of Manhattan, home of global health expert Jessica B. Martinez, had almost returned to normal. Trucks, stores, deliveries, and pedestrian traffic (with almost everyone masked) resembled prepandemic levels. In an interview, she assessed the long-term impact of the pandemic and the prospect of getting vaccinated against the virus.[17]

I STILL DON'T see my family, I still don't see my friends, I still don't go out for social reasons or to run errands. I don't travel for work. Nothing is the same. And it's because of the pandemic.

I'm scared for myself, so I don't want to get infected. And even though I know that now we have things like the monoclonal antibodies, and I know exactly how to get them, and I'm not terribly worried from a health perspective because I don't have any underlying comorbidities, I still don't want to get sick. And more importantly, I wouldn't want to be part of a chain of transmission. So no, nothing is the same.

How the pandemic has changed her

I had a pretty massive bout of insomnia for a while there and so I finally went and talked to a doctor about it. Prescribed a medicine that is non–habit forming, nonscary because that was a concern of mine. And so now I've been sleeping very well.

I've always been okay about dealing with stress. But I will say here and now I've realized that actually stress has gotten to me more than I thought over the past year. That was a bit of a shock.

I'm losing my hair. I've always had a lot of hair, and if I pull it back in a ponytail, the ponytail is thinner than it used to be. So I know that that's stress related.

I've gained weight because you try not to eat but even if you're just eating fruit, it's still more calories than you would normally eat.

I'm realizing that there have been stealth ways that I have been stressed without realizing that it's a much more insidious kind of stress. It's not the sort of gut punching, stomach twisting stress, it's more of the constant low-grade that has that impact.

My skin looks terrible. I'm breaking out. I'm like freaking forty-five years old and I have acne sometimes!

And I think I see the same in my husband. He is normally a very Zen person, but I have noticed that he's a little bit quicker now to anger or to get frustrated and that's unusual too. I hate to be clichéd and say that I'm stressed but I have to admit, I am.

I do try to be more active. We got an elliptical machine, so I try to get on that on a more regular basis. I try to force myself to do things that help to make my house a more comfortable environment, do the laundry, clean the house, cook. Maybe they're not enjoyable per se, but they break up the monotony. In the end I'm glad I got them done. They give me a bit of a sense of accomplishment.

Her new normal

I usually wake up around seven-thirty, eight o'clock. I go for a walk, try to wake myself up by doing a little bit of moving around. And then I spend a good two or three hours in the morning, New York time, just kind of catching up on emails. My day doesn't actually start in earnest until about noontime.

And then I start my workday. Lots and lots of meetings.

And my day usually goes until about seven or eight at night. And then I just kind of spend the rest of the evening with my husband, our cats, watch a bit of TV, read a bit. Pretty straightforward, kind of boring to be honest with you. You know, run some errands in between but nothing major.

The challenges of virtual meetings and work

I have to give a lot of props to the New York City broadband infrastructure. I haven't had significant problems. But I will say, it is tiring. In an effort to try to make sure that you're having that human connection, I personally feel like I have to be more expressive, I have to be more conscious about looking at the camera. There's an element of additional effort to make sure that those meetings go as well as they could go.

Work's been very frustrating for a lot of reasons. More frustrating than I think I would have imagined, which I think also is a huge contributor to stress.

I say no more to stuff at work. I don't raise my hand as readily as I used to for special projects and things like that.

I work in global health. And, I have been doing COVID work since last January. And it's been very rewarding in a lot of ways. But because of the nature of health care, in particular because of the nature of drug development, over the course of the year, there's been the realization that products fail, or promising therapeutics don't actually turn out to be as promising as you thought they were.

Her anticipation of the vaccine

Oh my god, I'm going to cry. I'm going to cry tears of joy and relief because the fact that there is a vaccine that's been made in a year, one year, is just amazing. Just scientifically speaking, it's just incredible, absolutely incredible.

But then also, to be able to not fear the virus, to be able to feel like I am vaccinated. I'll still wear my mask everywhere and I still will be conscious of being potentially a vector since we don't know whether or not it prevents asymptomatic infections, but just knowing that my family is safe, that I'm safe, that my husband is safe. When I managed to snag that appointment for my grandmother, within like thirty minutes of when my parents got their shots I cried. And I have a feeling I'm going to have a hard time not shedding tears of joy and relief when I get the vaccine.

I will see friends who are also vaccinated.

I will go to restaurants.

And I know that I would go and see friends who also hopefully would be similarly vaccinated. It would allow me to go out and just see people again. I know it sounds trite, but I really haven't seen people in a year, so it would be nice.

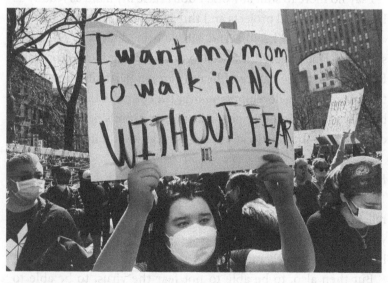

FIGURE 23

Demonstration against anti-Asian violence, Columbus Park, Chinatown, Manhattan, March 21, 2021. Photograph by Robert W. Snyder.

She reflects on how she is different from the person she was at the start of the pandemic and offers her thoughts on the storming of the US Capitol on January 6, 2021.

I don't think I've changed that much. I don't think I'm more cynical, but I do think I'm more worried. I think I'm a little bit less tolerant of other people and that makes me a little bit sad. There are people, either because of the way they behaved in the pandemic or because of the way that they reacted to what happened on the sixth, that I don't think I will ever be able to trust again. I'm a lot less tolerant of differences of opinion, quote unquote. So, in that sense I guess I'm a little bit less patient and more willing to draw a line in the sand. But otherwise, I don't think I'm that much different.

She has lost trust in both the people she encounters in her daily life and in the larger world.

I think it all sort of came to a head last year because I am of Hispanic background. My father is Hispanic, my mother is White, so I've been a mutt all my life. But I purposefully kept my last name Martinez, because my father only had daughters and it made him sad to think that he was the last of his line. Also I got married later in life and that's my name. I'm known that way. If I take my husband's name, I think people would probably think that I was White and so they have. I have had people say things in my presence who don't know my last name who look at me and don't necessarily see somebody who is Hispanic. I guess you could say I can pass. And they've said awful things.

So that's always been an issue, but it really became an issue now with Trump. I mean that happened from time to time, but I can count the times that it happened before Trump probably on one hand. Whereas now, it's a much more common occurrence, and of course that hits my parents, because my father is Mexican. And so, my mother has to see people act towards him in really horrible ways sometimes.

And then my husband is African American and now you have these people who were friends with my parents, some of whom are Hispanic and have experienced racism themselves because they're Hispanic, but are equally virulently racist against people who are Black.

It just really has laid bare a number of probably things that were just under the surface, but people were more polite. Or too polite to say anything about until now.

I have to admit, if I am not in New York, if I am out on Long Island where there's a pretty nasty strain of racism that's alive and where we have a weekend home, I worry about Will driving in a car by himself. I see people who are Caucasian and I worry, and I wonder. Are they Trump supporters, and will they see me or my husband as subhuman?

I never used to think about that. It never used to worry me. I never gave it a second thought, actually. And now I do. And that's awful. I hate that. I hate prejudging people and worrying about them just because of how they look, because that makes me like them.

Lexicon of the Pandemic

Pace High School students

By the spring of 2021, New Yorkers were so immersed in the pandemic that they had developed their own vocabulary to describe it. "Lexicon of the Pandemic" first appeared in Covid Class 2021, *a platform for students in David Rohlfing's English 12 class at Pace High School, a public school bordering Chinatown and the Lower East Side. Reflecting on the assignment that produced the lexicon, Rohlfing wrote, "High school students often think the authority of English class, the teacher and the educational institution are all designed to standardize language and their language. Though, of course, urban high school kids also understand the converse—that they are part of a vibrant culture that creates language and meaning of words. The pandemic gave us a sped-up and dramatic lesson in this, and it was easy and important to point it out to them. To give my students the job of recording these changes to language was also my attempt to empower them." Pace students, who come from all five boroughs and from many racial, ethnic, and economic backgrounds, compiled a list of words and phrases that came into use or took on new meanings during the pandemic.*[18]

A

anti-vaxxer someone who is against getting the COVID-19 vaccine.

antibody test a blood test to find antibodies from a previous COVID infection. "I think I had the COVID last March, because I lost my sense of smell for a week. I never got an antibody test, though."

asymptomatic somebody who has COVID-19 but isn't showing symptoms of the virus. "She was exposed to COVID but was asymptomatic."

asynchronous instruction a flexible form of teaching and learning in which lessons and work can be accessed and done at the students' leisure as long as it is done before the deadline given. "I'll go to the store for you since my classes are asynchronous today, I can worry about them later."

B

bandemic making money during the pandemic. "Pandemic turnt into a bandemic."

blended learning a style of education in which students learn via electronic and online media as well as traditional face-to-face teaching. "Due to the pandemic, students had to start blended learning."

C

clappy hour when New Yorkers went outside at 7:00 p.m. and clapped for health care workers during the height of the pandemic. "I brought my tambourine outside for clappy hour today and waved at my neighbors."

contact tracing the process of contacting all people who've had contact with someone who tested positive for COVID-19. "My mom got a new job during the pandemic doing contact tracing. She lets people know that they have been in contact with someone who has tested positive for the coronavirus and that they have to be quarantined."

COVID bubble people outside your household who you trust and feel comfortable being with safely during the pandemic. "My COVID bubble included my family and friends who I enjoyed my time with."

COVID party a gathering, at which the host typically has COVID-19, held to see how many people, if any, get COVID from the host. "I heard that two of the people that went to the COVID party last week are in really bad condition now."

Covidiot a person who doesn't wear their mask and doesn't social distance or follow simple COVID-19 protocols. "Don't be a Covidiot, stay at home if you feel sick."

COVID Karen a White woman who amplifies her privileges when it comes to exerting her opinions in reaction to the COVID virus. "I was greeted by a COVID Karen today at Target who was screaming, 'Stay six feet away!' at everyone in the cleaning aisle, even though she wasn't wearing a mask."

D

doomscrolling endlessly scrolling through social media for negativity and bad vibes. "No wonder I'm anxious and depressed, I just spent the past three hours doomscrolling."

double-vaxxed getting both shots of the vaccine. "Thank god, now that I'm double-vaxxed, hopefully I'm on track to making the world safer."

drive-thru testing getting a rapid COVID test from your car. "Before they let me in I had to get drive-thru tested."

E

essential worker someone who works in health care, transit, food, child care, or something that contributes to keeping the city running. "Essential workers risked their lives on the frontlines of the pandemic, so they had access to the vaccines first."

H

hybrid learning a combination of face-to-face learning and online learning. "When schools opened back up, students had to do hybrid learning."

hygiene theater a practice of taking hygiene measures such as wiping surfaces and wearing gloves and using hand sanitizer to give the feeling of improved safety from the virus. "It took about ten minutes to get into the store because of all the hygiene theater required."

I

immunocompromised a person's immune system's defenses are low, affecting its ability to fight off infections and diseases. People with this condition are at high risk of serious problems with COVID-19. Doctors have to care for immunocompromised patients so they advise them to wash their hands and keep their hygiene up.

L

lockdown a state of home isolation to keep from getting Covid. "During the COVID pandemic the city was put on lockdown and most public places were closed."

long hauler person who has gotten COVID-19 but still has symptoms or has not fully recovered after a long period of weeks or even months. "I can't believe Steve's still coughing and hasn't gained back his sense of smell, only taste! Hasn't it been like 4 weeks since he was diagnosed with COVID? What a long hauler!"

M

mask a protective mask that covers the nose and mouth to prevent the spread of COVID.

maskhole someone who does not care about the well-being of others and does not take the responsibility to put on a mask; also referred to someone who doesn't believe in the pandemic. "I ran into some maskhole while in the grocery store, I made sure to stay as far away as possible."

maskne acne from wearing a mask. "Jackson refused to turn on her video in Zoom class because she had a terrible case of maskne."

mute (unmute) when you pull yourself back from speaking during Zoom class. "After speaking with Mr. Rohlfing during class I put my audio on mute."

N

nonessential worker someone whose job isn't crucial to keep things running during a time like a pandemic or after a natural disaster. Many office workers in New York City were nonessential workers so they worked from home during the worst months of the pandemic.

P

personal protective equipment (PPE) essential workers and nonessential workers wear protective equipment to stay safe from contracting COVID-19. "I think we're running low on PPE again."

Q

quaranteens a not-so-nice way to describe the generation that is stuck living their teenage years indoors during quarantine. "I hate being a quaranteen, I'm never going to enjoy my senior year—no prom, no formal graduation!!"

R

remote learning the temporary move from in-person face-to-face learning to learning online from home. "The school called and said we were switching to remote learning."

The Rona the term we use to describe the coronavirus. "Put your mask on, Rona outside."

S

shelter in place find a safe location indoors and stay there until you are given an "all clear" or told it's safe to come out. "We had to shelter in place when coronavirus hit New York City."

social distancing the practice of staying more than six feet away from another person to decrease the risk of being in contact with someone who may be infectious.

social isolation when someone isolates themselves from society, usually because they have been exposed to someone with COVID or they have tested positive for COVID themselves. People do this so they don't spread the virus. "Last week I had to go through a social isolation because I tested positive for COVID."

stimmy the stimulus check that American people received for financial help. "Yo, my stimmy came in, let's go to Miami!"

superspreader events that cause COVID-19 to spread fast to a large group of people; a person who spreads the virus to a massive amount of people typically in the crowd or at a social gathering. "Someone's having another superspreader party." "Stay away from that dude, you can tell he's a superspreader."

swab a material used by health workers for taking samples from the nose for a COVID test; the act of taking a sample to test for COVID-19. The swabbing is then repeated on the other side of the nose to make sure enough material is collected. "As she put the nasal swab up my nose, it felt as if I was going to sneeze."

T

test the process in which people can know whether they carry the COVID virus or not. "My mom went with her friend to get a test at CityMD."

U

unemployment people who lost their jobs received money to help pay bills. "Yo, did you get unemployment today because you've been out of work for about two weeks now?"

V

vaccine hesitant a person who delays or refuses to take the COVID-19 vaccination. "Mr. Jones was vaccine hesitant until he had to return to the school."

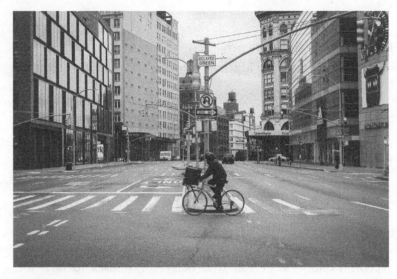

FIGURE 24
Before vaccines: Houston Street in lower Manhattan, March 25, 2020. Photograph courtesy of the City of New York.

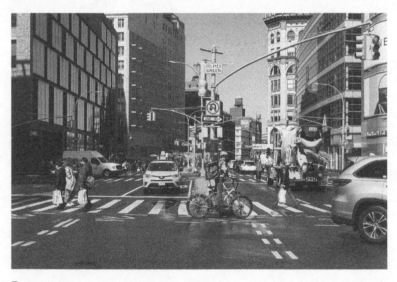

FIGURE 25
After vaccines: Houston Street in lower Manhattan, April 12, 2022. Photograph courtesy of the City of New York.

Eating Bitterness

Mackenzie Kwok

Mackenzie Kwok, a Chinese American folklorist and singer-songwriter based in Brooklyn, New York, turned to music to process pandemic experiences that included violence against Asian Americans. As she noted, well after vaccines reduced the deadliness of COVID-19, racist violence threatened Asian Americans.[19]

MY FAVORITE SUBWAY station in New York is the Canal Street Q station. I love that it is the first stop in Manhattan on the ride from Brooklyn, after crossing the Manhattan Bridge where everyone catches their breath as they look out the window. I love that it's in Chinatown, right around the corner from vendors selling knock-off Louis Vuitton purses. I love the store directly up the stairs, the window adorned with bags of all sizes in the shape of chickens. I love the sign on the window that reads, "Look at all my chickens."

But the Canal Street station also has me on edge lately. I don't recall the last time I peered over the platform edge to see if the train was on the way. Not since Michelle Go was pushed to her death in Times Square in 2022. Not since an Asian friend from my running club mentioned that he'd had a knife pulled on him at that station. Not since spa workers in Atlanta were killed. Not since a man uttered "*ni hao,* sexy," to me on a dark walk home one night.

Let me be clear: I don't feel personally targeted. I do not feel that there are racist men out to attack me. I do not even live in a historically Asian neighborhood where many of these anti-Asian hate crimes frequently take place. Still, I have learned to keep away from the edge of the subway platform, to dress boyishly when I am out alone, to keep quiet so I do not stir the pot.

In Chinese, there is a phrase, 吃苦 (*chi ku*). It means "to eat bitterness," to endure hardship, to carry on, to persevere. My great-grandparents, Kao Tsao-Yuan and Loh Mei-Chun, fled Shanghai for Hong Kong in 1949 before settling in the Bronx in 1960. They crossed through Ellis Island amidst intense immigration restrictions from Asian countries. Leaving Shanghai was their bitterness to eat, as was navigating a new country.

In February 2020, I went to a comedy show in Brooklyn. During a moment of audience interaction with edgy humor, the host asked what my ethnicity is. I said "Chinese." She said "Stay away from me. Coronavirus made me racist." I didn't know what to do in front of an audience that, to be fair, was also getting roasted. I didn't say anything, but I pretended to cough. I did not stick up for myself; I just went along with it. This, to me, was eating bitterness. By not resisting the joke, I was swallowing my discomfort through a joke and a smile.

I eat bitterness in the Canal Street subway station when I take care to stay by the wall, or stand toward the middle of the platform. I eat bitterness when men in cars comment on my body, and I stay silent, hoping they'll leave. I eat bitterness feeling that I am safe while wondering if I will be singled out as a lone Asian woman to the wrong person with hungry eyes.

Sometimes, when I tell people about being followed, they will tell me I am strong. That's what eating bitterness is, after all, a sign of grit and strength. But to me, being called strong is the most bitter taste to chew on. I do not stay silent out of strength; I do so out of protection for myself. I do so out of anxiety, even fear.

I wrote a song for Annie Lanzillotto's *Tell Me a Story* salon, a virtual talk show that began during lockdown. Annie, an artist and community activist, invited me and other young women to share pieces for an episode called "The Orb of F— Off: Girls' Bodies/ Public Spaces." During a brainstorm session, Annie asked, "What is breaking your heart most today?" I said, "Being called a strong woman." Eating bitterness and being told I'm noble for it. I wrote this song called "The Bitterness I Eat." The first verse goes like this:

I'm not strong, it's just I have to be
Thirteen years of mediating
Man, it's getting heavy.
What do you want me to say
When I'm followed down the street?
Thank you for the bitterness I eat?

There is much bitterness now, following the Sunset Park subway attack and more deaths in Chinatown. As New Yorkers are well aware, life goes on not because we are brave, but because we have no other choice. Sliding my hand into my pocket and feeling for the sharp edges of my brass knuckles lets me feel relief when I am on edge. So does keeping away from the end of the train platform, or covering myself with baggy clothing at night. I don't want to live in fear, but I have these little lines of defense, just in case.

I pray that the Chinatown community, that Asian American elders, parents, young adults, and children, are not called "strong" for going about life after hate crimes. We are unsure and afraid. "Text me when you get home" has an additional layer of concern to it. I pray that our community is met with the gentleness and softness we deserve instead of being called "resilient."

We can eat bitterness, but I am tired of it. I would like something sweet. I would like to be able to lean over to see if the Q train is coming again.

The Island of Pandemica

Steve Zeitlin

By April 2021, when the folklorist Steve Zeitlin wrote "The Island of Pandemica," the vaccine was already in use and the culture of fear had eased enough for him to end this poem on a semi-hopeful note.[20]

On the island of Pandemica
we struggled, isolated and alone,
surrounded by contaminated waters

disturbed by those
who accidentally dipped their toes
and went under
or who, stranded in the poison rain,
suffocated in a bed alone,
their families torn asunder.

Till, one year later, we flexed our vaccinated muscles
and started swimming towards dry land.
Let us pray that for
the younger generation,
children of the plague,
Pandemica might be a place to which we traveled—
a distant, foreign land.

8

Reflections, 2023

On May 11, 2023, the Biden administration ended the COVID-19 emergency declarations that had enabled measures like the distribution of free COVID-19 tests. Although subvariants of the coronavirus remained in circulation, with vaccines and evolving medical knowledge these were far more manageable than earlier forms of the virus. But this did not mean the end of thinking about the pandemic.[1]

From the earliest days of the pandemic, New Yorkers tried to make sense of what they were going through. Some turned to religion, some relied on family and friends, and some worked for political change. Many simply wanted to forget COVID-19 and get back to what they called "the before times."

In the oral histories and first-person narratives that I read, people spoke memorably about the future. They yearned not just for a world without COVID-19, but for a world reborn where the hard knowledge gained during COVID-19 would be applied to building a better city and country, with strong support for public health, so that no one would ever again have to face anything like the pandemic.

Whether those high hopes are realized will depend on how we remember the COVID-19 pandemic in New York City. One possibility is that people will simply forget about it—much as they forgot about the flu pandemic of 1918, which took an estimated

50 million or more lives worldwide, killed some thirty thousand in New York City alone, and left no imprint in public memorials or collective memory in New York or the United States. Even though scientists studied the flu epidemic and historians wrote about it, most memories of the 1918 flu were banished to private realms of grieving and loss, sorely limiting the chance of any public and collective effort to learn lessons that would help us avoid repeating past mistakes.[2]

As unfathomable as it seemed in the spring of 2020, forgetting COVID-19 now seems much more plausible, much more human even—the understandable reaction to a traumatic event that most people would like to put behind them. But maybe we can do better. If New Yorkers look squarely at how people suffered from crippling inequalities, remember with empathy all who worked to help the city through its ordeal, and recognize that the health of each of us is inseparable from the health of all of us, then New York City's passage through the pandemic will not have been in vain.

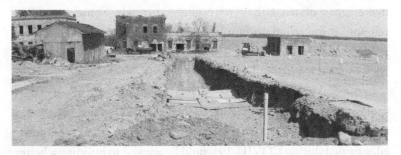

Figure 26
May 2, 2021: A mass burial on Hart Island, the final resting place in New York City for the indigent, the unclaimed, the unidentified, and the stillborn. The island has been the site of mass burials since 1872, but images of coffins and trenches there during the pandemic left many New Yorkers feeling that their city was in a deep crisis. Photograph by Alon Sicherman and Sean Vegezzi for The Hart Island Project.

Learning How to Talk to People

Dave Crenshaw

In May 2023 Dave Crenshaw reflected on what he had learned working to help his neighbors in Washington Heights survive the pandemic.[3]

EVERYTHING IS ABOUT confidence. You have to learn how to talk to people. And the way you talk to them is like they're all your neighbors. What they think is important. What they think matters.

When you're talking with seniors you're gonna listen to all their stories. They want someone to talk to. Isolation is damaging. They need someone to hear their stories.

People should not be treated like patients. We should be treated like neighbors.

Whenever something went wrong, we were brainstorming how not to let that happen again. We didn't want to see people walk away frustrated, that very rarely happened. But anyone who tells you it never happened is a liar.

We built up a network of people we could count on, people you could trust, people you could work with.

The whole key to surviving this was who had correct information. And could you deliver it to people.

It was never just me. It was always a team effort. The Mailman interns and the Black Health interns and my alumni from Team Dreamers and PS 128, we just worked together.

Strength in the Long Run

Richard Brea

Richard Brea, commander of the 46th Precinct in the West Bronx during the early months of the pandemic, retired from the NYPD in June 2020 and went to work in the security industry. In April 2023, he assessed the long-term impact of the pandemic on New York City.[4]

I DO KNOW that if, God forbid, there is another pandemic, the world is more prepared to handle it. I think that there's been a lot of lessons learned from COVID-19. We can say that some things worked well, and perhaps other things didn't. This was a trial run.

I think we did okay. There were some unfortunate losses. But I think in the end, it will make us all stronger.

"We Were Here"

Re'gan Weal

Re'gan Weal, a bus operator, reflects on the pandemic.[5]

IT WAS ROUGH. It was a sad time. We lost a lot of people here. A lot of people feared for their lives. You had some people who were crying, you had people who were depressed. It was a rough time, you had to make the best of it.

Transit has their rules, but sometimes I feel they don't consider us. I just think they should recognize us more, they should consider us a little more, as well because sometimes it seems like they care more about the public and the public doesn't care about us either.

It's not over, but I'm glad we're not where we were in 2020. I'm glad we're not seeing people drop like flies anymore. Because that's what it felt like, every time we turned around someone was dead. And it could have been you at any time.

We were here. We got you from point A to point B. It was a ghost town here. But we were still up and down the streets. The trains were still running. We were here. We were risking our lives, our families, while everyone else was home. I just really would like people to remember that we were here.

Remembering Sacrifices and Losses

Veronica E. Fletcher

In February 2023, Veronica E. Fletcher reflected on her late husband Joseph Trevor Fletcher, a transit worker who died of COVID-19, and all the workers whose labor kept things functioning in New York, the United States, and the world.[6]

ONE OF THE things that I hope that we can't forget in our country, and throughout the world, are the sacrifices of people who lost their lives to help us get through this time. There are doctors, there are nurses. There are truck drivers that sacrificed their lives to deliver goods and services. There are grocery stores employees and pharmacists who sacrificed to serve others. There are police officers, firefighters, MTA workers, there are essential workers throughout this country who lost their lives, sacrificed their lives, to keep our country moving, to keep the world moving.

As we celebrate getting through it's imperative that we also acknowledge the sacrifices that were made by people to get us through. And that we also remember that there are people who are living with loss.

I know that my late husband hasn't been forgotten by the lives that he touched. He sacrificed his life for people that will never know his name. People that will never know what the sacrifice entailed. He went and did his job and made sure that people could continue living their lives, could continue saving lives. And that was in essence who he was, a generous, generous, selfless, giving individual who died as he lived as a hero.

The Momentum and Tumult of Discovery

Steven Palmer

Steven Palmer, a physician assistant at Columbia Medical Center, considers how his understanding of COVID-19 has evolved since the spring of 2020.[7]

WHEN HIV HAPPENED in the early 1980s with people not knowing what it was and how it worked, there was a whole evolution of scientific and medical understanding that ultimately pushed the world of medicine and science forward. Necessity is the mother of invention. And I think that is happening as a result of COVID as well. And also because of long COVID.

We're not at the absolute beginning stages of the momentum of discovery, but we're still in the infancy or toddler moment.

When something like this hits, you can have all the best scientists and clinicians and virologists in the world and there's no way to get it right immediately. It takes time to try and figure out the trajectory of these viruses and what they're going to cause, and how to deal with them.

Everybody is involved in the tumult of discovery. I look back at the whole thing, and I just recognize that there's no way to take the smartest of everything and have it go smoothly. It's always going to be a rocky ride.

Facing the future

Long COVID is a real thing. This whole thing of brain fog is real. And POTS, which is Postural Orthostatic Tachycardia Syndrome; Dysautonomia, which is the autonomic nervous system having been affected, all of these things are real. The worsening of irritable bowel syndrome in people who have irritable bowel syndrome.

Long COVID is real, and we're gonna need money for that. We're learning more and more and we have a number of people who have come out of long COVID, but there's a lot of people who are still suffering. We have a ways to go with studies and research to figure this out.

These folks want their lives back. They want this over. Right now we're able to help people who haven't come out of it completely, but may feel stuck in their recovery. The relief of being better than you had been is still met with the natural impatience of wanting to be back to your pre-COVID life. That's our task now—to figure out how to get there.

"Look Out for Each Other"

Keerthan Thiyagarajah

Keerthan Thiyagarajah from Jackson Heights, Queens, looks back on the pandemic and what can be learned from it.[8]

REFLECTING BACK ON the pandemic, I think my biggest takeaway is to just love each other, no matter who you are, Asian, Black, White, it doesn't matter what you are. Just learn to love and care about one another. At the end of the day, we're all humans. We all need to care for each other. Look out for each other. The biggest takeaway for me especially was to just help people, especially people that can't help themselves.

New York, it's one of those cities where people kind of mind their own business, and they kind of just don't look out for each other, but at the end of the day New Yorkers will band together.

We're all New Yorkers. We all have that New York tough style, it's bred in us whether we grew up here or we moved here. It's ingrained in you to be New York tough, New York strong.

We should be our own leaders. We should set that standard. New Yorkers are leaders in their own way. That's why when we don't have that leader, we embody it within ourselves to be the leaders that we need in our communities to help each other.

Conclusion

COVID-19 battered New York City's reputation as a can-do city prepared for any emergency. Despite the city's many renowned hospitals and respected institutions dedicated to public health, COVID-19 claimed 46,426 lives from March 2020 to June 2024 and reduced the life expectancy of New Yorkers citywide, especially among Blacks and Hispanics. Each death had its own ripple effect, and even if you were one of the fortunate New Yorkers who did not lose anyone close to you, eventually you heard of people in the distant corners of your human ecosystem who died.

As the sociologist Paul Starr has observed, "The American response to COVID-19 has encapsulated an era when a nation that has always thought of itself as a success has had to confront the possibility that its luck had run out." His observation applies equally to the city of New York.[1]

Every level of government—federal, state, and local—failed to some degree. President Trump abdicated responsibility. The mayor and governor, fearful of the adverse economic impact of strong public health measures, ignored or contradicted the advice of the city's health department—delaying the city's response to COVID-19 while the disease raced through the population. The city's best-funded private hospitals barely held on, while the public hospitals that served the city's poor faced catastrophic conditions.

By the standards of the neoliberal era that preceded the pandemic, with its emphasis on for-profit medicine and market-based modes of planning, New York City had a world class medical system equipped to provide cutting-edge treatment for chronic diseases like cancer. What it needed in the pandemic was a more social democratic system prepared to treat rich and poor equally well in an epidemic driven by a communicable virus. To frame it in terms of the city's mayors, it needed less of Giuliani and more of LaGuardia.

Across the United States, in debates over mandates, masking, and vaccination, the sense of solidarity among Americans was torn almost to the vanishing point. The pandemic left New York City and the United States with much work to do building trust

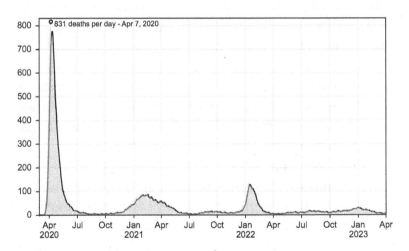

FIGURE 27
Deaths per day and rolling averages in New York City. Chart: BetaNYC. Data: New York City Department of Health and Mental Hygiene

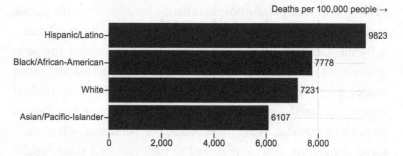

FIGURE 28
Death rates by race and ethnicity in New York City. Chart: BetaNYC. Data:
New York City Department of Health and Mental Hygiene.

and a sense of common purpose among people who will someday
face again the threats of health emergencies and natural disasters.
This will be difficult, especially in a world where so much work is
virtual and the digital world emphasizes niche markets and nar-
rowly tailored personal satisfactions over broadly shared experiences. As the pandemic reminded us, city life is characterized by
the interdependence of people who are strangers to each other.
The stories of friends, families, neighbors, and workers who pulled
together in the pandemic are inspiring, but they are the stories of
women and men in relatively small groups who built on existing
connections. Future challenges will require us to bond on a larger
scale if we are to be effective.[2]

If New Yorkers and Americans are to remember COVID-19 in
a way that prepares us to do better when the next disaster hits us,
we need to understand not only the city's failures but also what
New Yorkers did best in the pandemic: connect with their friends,
families, neighbors, and workmates and forge bonds of solidarity
that enabled them to help one another. Such solidarity sustained
people in the darkest days of the pandemic and enabled New

Yorkers to successfully engage in social distancing, bending the curve of infections and deaths so that casualties plummeted from some eight hundred deaths a day to a more manageable level by the end of May 2020. Solidarity among workers also sustained a growth in labor union activity in the city and nationwide that was one of the notable occurrences of the pandemic era. While it is too early to pronounce the neoliberal order finished, if the United States is ever to regain the broader level of prosperity and equality that characterized it from the 1930s to the 1970s, a reinvigorated labor movement and strong unions will be essential.

While the most public and physical manifestation of this solidarity was the 7:00 p.m. cheers, many others, unheralded, deserve recognition: Elizabeth Petrillo, the supermarket cashier who became "like a therapist to her customers"; Ralph Rolle, the entrepreneur who made his restaurant as safe as possible for his staff and customers; and Maribel Gonzalez Christianson, the bar owner who realized that her deliveries of food orders were sometimes the one episode of human contact that her customers had in a long time. Even without face-to-face contact, people found ways to reach out to one another in emails and texts, in Facebook posts and phone calls. People used Zoom for everything from cocktail parties to classes to public meetings. Creative young producers turned Zoom into a tool to produce panel discussions and interviews that recovered the best promises of the early days of public television as a forum for civic engagement.

To be sure there were divisions, such as the disagreements over the importance and efficacy of masks. Mask wearers, generally Democrats and supporters of governmental public health efforts, thought of themselves as protecting themselves and protecting others. Antimaskers—likely to be Trump supporters, Republicans, or libertarians—valued individual freedom above all and dismissed the value of masking. Maskers could look at antimaskers and see libertarianism run amok, while antimaskers saw in masked New Yorkers the coercive power of the state. Each discerned in the other arrogance and unwarranted certainty. But the brave and generous conduct of ordinary New Yorkers toward friends, neighbors, families, and even strangers helped the city survive the crisis.

If the importance of acts of solidarity among ordinary people is one insight of this book, the value of a socially conscious

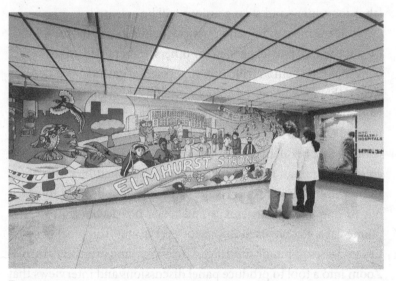

FIGURE 29
Elmhurst Strong, a mural by Luis Fernando Lechón in Elmhust Hospital Center, in Queens—the "epicenter of the epicenter." The mural, unveiled in 2020, is one of twenty-six at public hospitals and health care facilities in New York City funded by the Community Mural Project of the Laurie M. Tisch Illumination Fund for the NYC Health + Hospitals Community Mural Project. Photo by Nicholas Knight, courtesy of the Laurie M. Tisch Illumination Fund

Luis Fernando Lechón: "In the mural, we can see a community strengthened by solidarity. The mural also expresses gratitude to all health workers, acknowledging all the effort and dedication they give every day. . . . Elmhurst is a diverse multicultural, multilingual neighborhood."

professionalism in public health emergencies is another. Nurses, doctors, first responders, transit workers, and EMTs all confronted the crisis with a professionalism grounded in mutual obligations to one another and to the public they serve.

It is embodied in the memories of EMT Phil Suarez, who said he couldn't live with himself if he abandoned his work during COVID-19; in the police commander Richard Brea telling his officers who were reluctant to enter a home infected with COVID-19 that they promised to face danger when they swore an oath to become a police officer; in Patricia Tiu, going online with video reports from "the gates of hell" to steel her fellow nurses against the pandemic; and Re'gan Weal, driving a bus daily in the depths of the pandemic despite all dangers of infection.

The pandemic was a tragedy in New York City, but to fail to learn from it would be a tragedy twice over. If we are to learn anything from the COVID-19 years in New York City, the best place to begin is with the words of the people who drove ambulances, cared for patients, punched cash registers, drove buses, ran trains, and faced death daily so that others might live.

Remembering their stories and sacrifices is the way to prepare for a better future.

Acknowledgments

M y first thanks go to the people who sat for interviews, wrote first-person narratives or poems, conducted interviews, and took photographs that are shared in this book. All are recognized individually on our contributors page. I am also grateful for the data visualizations of BetaNYC and for the photograph of Luis Fernando Lechón's mural at Elmhurst Hospital Center in Queens taken by Nicholas Knight. Collectively, their work embodies the strength, humanity, and resourcefulness that New Yorkers brought to the challenges of COVID-19.

The majority of the interviews, narratives, and poems presented in this book were first collected in oral history projects, archival projects, and poetry projects in New York City. My thanks go to Ryan Hagen, Mary Marshall Clark, and Amy Starecheski of The NYC COVID-19 Oral History, Narrative, and Memory Project at Columbia University; Mark Nowak of the Worker Writers School; Natalie Milbrodt of Queens Memory; Thomas Cleary, librarian/archivist and assistant professor at LaGuardia Community College; Molly Rosner, director of Education Programs at the LaGuardia and Wagner Archives at LaGuardia Community College; Susan Smith-Peter, professor of history at the College of Staten Island and founder of the Lockdown Staten Island project; Steve Zeitlin and Seth Schonberg of City Lore; Claire Solomon Nisen, manager of Lasting Impressions at DOROT; Mark Naison and the students and faculty who worked on the Bronx COVID-19 Oral History Project at Fordham University; Rick Luftglass of the Healing Walls Project at the Laurie M. Tisch Illumination Fund; and Miriam Deutch, associate professor and director of the Open Educational Resources Initiative at the Brooklyn College Library, who served as cofounder and director of the Brooklyn College Journal of the Plague Year COVID-19 Archive. Ellen Noonan, clinical associate professor of history and director of the archives and public history program at New York University; and Peter Aigner, director of the Gotham Center for New York City History at the CUNY Graduate Center, created websites that helped historians, archivists, and documentarians grapple with the challenges of COVID-19.

Historians David Rosner, Janet Golden, and Josh Brown helped me think historically about the pandemic. I also learned much from the participants in the Living New Deal panel "COVID-19, the Great Depression, and the Battle between Memory and Forgetting," which was ably moderated by Margaret Crane. Participants included Dave Chokshi, MD; Sharon Musher, associate professor of history at Stockton University; and Karen Kruse Thomas of the Johns Hopkins Bloomberg School of Public Health. (I could not participate because I had COVID-19.)

Gracia Brown and Brendan Reynolds insightfully read scores of interviews and helped me winnow them down. Jessica Siegel's research directed me to valuable pieces, including the work of David Rohlfing's students at Pace High School. Elaine Abelson and Paul Sternberger helped me make some difficult choices in selecting photographs for illustrations, and Fritz Umbach helped me work through drafts of the book's introduction and more. Kristen La Follette helped me compare and understand coping strategies during the pandemic and the Great Depression. Chris Herrmann helped me with statistics on crime. Mary Marshall Clark helped me think through issues regarding oral history, memory, and the work of nurses. Ada Huang, MD, read drafts of my chapter introductions.

Al Howard and Ron Grele introduced me to oral history. I have been grateful for their teaching and friendship ever since.

Reporting in the *New York Times*, THE CITY, and *Gothamist* helped me navigate the pandemic as a resident and a researcher and affirmed the importance of local journalism in a global city.

This book was produced during my term as Manhattan Borough historian to document New York City's passage through a crisis and leave a record of the COVID-19 pandemic for future generations. I am grateful to Gale Brewer for appointing me Borough Historian during her term as Manhattan Borough President and to her successor, Mark Levine, for continuing my appointment.

As in every book I have written, I have been inspired by writers and authors who have come before me. The COVID-19 pandemic is the biggest domestic crisis to hit the United States since the Great Depression; in my work on the pandemic, I was inspired by the writers and editors of the Federal Writers Project, who worked to weave together a divided and suffering country in the 1930s. In *Strange Defeat: A Statement of Evidence Written in 1940,* the French historian, soldier, and Resistance member Marc Bloch sought to understand how France was defeated so badly in 1940 and what it needed to do to revive itself as a republic. The United States needs a similar examination. George Orwell's essay "The Lion and the Unicorn: Socialism and the English Genius," written in the early days of World War II, argued that to win the war England needed to become a more democratic and more egalitarian country. I have learned from all these works, and I think they have something to teach other Americans in the shadow of COVID-19.

Two peer reviewers engaged by Cornell University Press offered questions and suggestions that strengthened the book in the home stretch. Any errors that remain despite the suggestions of all these good readers and advisers are my own fault.

Michael McGandy, formerly an editor at Cornell University Press and now director of the University of South Carolina Press, offered valuable advice in the early days of planning this book. He was followed at Cornell by Mahinder Kingra, who handed the book off to Meagan Levinson, editorial director of the Three Hills imprint at Cornell University Press. Meagan's sharp suggestions and collegial encouragement improved the book and sustained my morale in the home stretch. I am also grateful for the help I received from the rest of the Cornell team: Acquisitions Assistant India Miraglia, copy editor Jack Rummel, Assistant Managing Editor Karen Laun, Production Coordinator Kate LeBoff, and, in marketing, Alex Vlahov and Alfredo Gutierrez Rios.

As with every book I have written, Peter Eisenstadt was a great source of historical and editorial suggestions. My wife, the journalist Clara Hemphill, provided superior editorial advice and was an excellent companion in the long months and years of the COVID-19 pandemic.

Notes

Introduction

1. Trends and Totals page of NYC Health at https://www.nyc.gov/site/doh/covid/covid-19-data-totals.page.

2. David P. Fidler, *SARS, Governance, and the Globalization of Disease* (London: Palgrave Macmillan, 2004), 71, 99–105.

3. Joseph S. Lieber, Sandra Opdycke, and David Rosner, "Public Health," in *Encyclopedia of New York City*, 2nd ed., ed. Kenneth T. Jackson (New Haven: Yale University Press, 2010), 1048–52.

4. On the death of social democratic New York City in the fiscal crisis, see Joshua B. Freeman, *Working-Class New York: Life and Labor Since World War II* (New York: New Press, 2000), 270–83; Kim Phillips-Fein, *Fear City: New York's Fiscal Crisis and the Rise of Austerity Politics* (New York: Metropolitan Books, 2017), 304–16; and Jonathan Soffer, *Ed Koch and the Rebuilding of New York* (New York: Columbia University Press, 2020), 3–4, 191–203, 400–401. On the general problems of delivering health care in New York, see Bruce F. Berg, *Healing Gotham: New York City's Public Health Policies for the Twenty-First Century* (Baltimore: Johns Hopkins University Press, 2015), 16–17 and 26–30. On broad patterns of inequality in New York City hospitals, see George Aumoithe, "Dismantling the Safety-Net Hospital: The Construction of 'Underutilization' and Scarce Public Hospital Care," *Journal of Urban History* 49, no. 6 (2023): 1282–84, 1285–88, 1291, 1295–97, 1300–1301; and on the shortage of beds early in the pandemic, Carl Campanile, Julia Marsh, Bernadette Hogan, and Nolan Hicks, "New York Has Thrown Away 20,000 Hospital Beds, Complicating Coronavirus Fight," *New York Post*, March 17, 2020, updated March 28, 2020, https://nypost.com/2020/03/17/new-york-has-thrown-away-20000-hospital-beds-complicating-coronavirus-fight.

5. Figures on the death toll of the flu of 1918 in New York City vary. Francesco Aimone's figure of thirty thousand includes deaths from both flu and pneumonia, a common combination of illnesses that contributed to the deadly nature

of the flu. See Francesco Aimone, "The 1918 Influenza Epidemic in New York City: A Review of the Public Health Response," *Public Health Reports* 125 (2010): 71–79. Useful books on the flu epidemic of 1918 include Alfred W. Crosby, *America's Forgotten Pandemic: The Influenza of 1918* (New York: Cambridge University Press, 2003); and Laura Spinney, *Pale Rider: The Spanish Flu and How it Changed the World* (New York: Public Affairs, 2017).

6. The most important collections for this book were the NYC COVID-19 Oral History, Narrative, and Memory Project at https://incite.columbia. edu/covid19-oral-history-project; Lockdown Staten Island Collection at https://covid-19archive.org/s/lockdown-staten-island/page/welcome; Fordham University's The Bronx COVID-19 Oral History Project at https://www.thebronx covid19oralhistoryproject.com/; the Queens Memory COVID-19 Project at https://library.qc.cuny.edu/blog/queens-memory-covid-19-project/; Brooklyn College Journal of the Plague Year at https://covid-19archive.org/s/brooklyncollege/ page/welcome; and the Museum of the City of New York's "New York Responds Online" at https://www.mcny.org/new-york-responds-online. The folklorists of City Lore are at https://citylore.org/. For a website documenting COVID-related historical projects see, at the website of the Gotham Center for New York City History, the "COVID-NYC Documentary Project" at https://www.gothamcenter.org/ covidnyc-documentary-project and, at New York University, Historians Respond to COVID-19 athttps://wp.nyu.edu/covid19histories/category/collecting/oralhis tory/.

7. The phrase "alone together" dates to the song "Alone Together," lyrics by Howard Dietz and music by Arthur Schwartz. The song was introduced in 1932 in the Broadway musical *Flying Colors*.

8. Paul Fussell, *Class: A Guide to the American Status System* (New York: Summit Books, 1983), 25–26.

9. "Trends and Totals," NYC Health, at https://www.nyc.gov/site/doh/covid/ covid-19-data-totals.page; and "COVID-19 Update for the United States," Centers for Disease Control and Prevention, at https://covid.cdc.gov/covid-data-tracker/#datatracker-home.

10. Rebecca Solnit, *A Paradise Built in Hell: The Extraordinary Communities That Arise in Disasters* (New York: Penguin Books, 2009), Kindle 2–3.

11. Vaclav Havel, *Summer Meditations* (New York: Knopf, 1992), 8–9.

1. Early Days, Winter 2020

1. See "At Novel Coronavirus Briefing, Governor Cuomo Announces State is Partnering with Hospitals to Expand Novel Coronavirus Testing Capacity in New York," March 2, 2020, Albany, NY, at https://www.governor.ny.gov/news/video-audio-photos-rush-transcript-novel-coronavirus-briefing-governor-cuomo-announces-state.

2. Trends and totals: https://www.nyc.gov/site/doh/covid/covid-19-data-totals.page.

3. The COVID Crisis Group, *Lessons From the Covid War: An Investigative Report* (New York: PublicAffairs, 2023), 30. On the importance of thinking about epidemics and disasters historically, see David Rosner, ed., *Hives of Sickness: Public Health and Epidemics in New York City* (New York: Museum of the City of New York/Rutgers University Press, 1995); and Andy Horowitz, *Katrina: A History, 1915-2015* (Cambridge: Harvard University Press, 2020).

4. Daniel T. Rodgers, *The Age of Fracture* (Cambridge: Harvard University Press, 2012); The COVID Crisis Group, *Lessons From the Covid War*, 24–26, 119, 127–28; and Lawrence Wright, *The Plague Year: America in the Time of Covid* (New York: Alfred A. Knopf, 2021), 14–18; and Paul Starr, "Reckoning with National Failure: The Case of Covid," *Liberties* 1, no. 3 (spring 2021): 73–75, 77–80. For Trump speculating on cures, see Daniel Funke, "In Context: What Donald Trump Said about Disinfectant, Sun, and Coronavirus," *POLITIFACT*, April 24, 2020, https://www.politifact.com/article/2020/apr/24/context-what-donald-trump-said-about-disinfectant-/. For Trump's attacks on critics, see Lisa Friedman and Brad Plumer, "Trump's Response to Virus Reflects a Long Disregard for Science," *New York Times*, April 28, 2020, https://www.nytimes.com/2020/04/28/climate/trump-coronavirus-climate-science.html; and Quint Forgey, "Trump Attacks Second Democratic Governor over Coronavirus Criticism," *POLITICO*, March 19, 2020, https://www.politico.com/news/2020/03/09/trump-attacks-second-democratic-governor-over-coronavirus-criticism-124216.

5. See Benjamin M. Althouse, Brendan Wallace, Brendan Case, Samuel V. Scarpino, Antoine Allard, Andrew M. Berdahl, Easton R. White, and Laurent Hebert-Dufresne, "The Unintended Consequences of Inconsistent Pandemic Control Policies," National Library of Medicine (2020), https://www.ncbi.nlm.nih.gov/pmc/articles/PMC7457624/; and Karen DeSalvo, Bob Hughes, Mary Bassett, Georges Benjamin, Michael Fraser, Sandro Galea, and J. Nadine Gracia, "Public Health COVID-19 Impact Assessment: Lessons Learned and Compelling Needs," *NAM PERSPECTIVES*, April 7, 2021, https://www.ncbi.nlm.nih.gov/pmc/articles/PMC8406505/.

6. Gary Gerstle, *The Rise and Fall of the Neoliberal Order: America and the World in the Free Market Era* (New York: Oxford University Press, 2022), 5–6, 161, 173, 207–27, 241–67.

7. Berg, *Healing Gotham*, 16–18, 21, 25–30, 247–49; and the essays in Joshua B. Freeman, ed., *City of Workers, City of Struggle: How Labor Movements Changed New York* (New York: Columbia University Press, 2019).

8. Michael Schwirtz, "One Rich N.Y. Hospital Got Warren Buffett's Help, One Got Duct Tape," *New York Times*, April 26, 2929, https://www.nytimes.com/2020/04/26/nyregion/coronavirus-new-york-university-hos

pital.html; Brian M. Rosenthal, Joseph Goldstein, Sharon Otterman, and Sheri Fink, "Why Surviving the Virus Might Come Down to Which Hospital Admits You," *New York Times*, July 1, 2020, https://www.nytimes.com/2020/07/01/nyregion/Coronavirus-hospitals.html; Amanda Dunker and Elizabeth Benjamin, "How Structural Inequalities in New York's Health Care System Exacerbate Health Disparities During the COVID-19 Pandemic: A Call for Equitable Reform," New York: Community Service Society, June 4, 2020.

9. Dunker and Benjamin, "Structural Inequalities in New York's Health Care System," 1–2, 5; Clare Malone, "New York's Inequalities Are Fueling COVID-19," 538, April 10, 2020, https://fivethirtyeight.com/features/wealth-and-race-have-always-divided-new-york-covid-19-has-only-made-things-worse/; and Elise Gould and Heidi Shierholz, "Not Everybody Can Work from Home," Working Economic Blog, Economic Policy Institute, March 19, 2020, https://www.epi.org/blog/black-and-hispanic-workers-are-much-less-likely-to-be-able-to-work-from-home/.

10. Hannah Kuchler and Andrew Edgecliffe-Johnson, "How New York's Missteps Let Covid-19 Overwhelm the US," *Financial Times*, October 22, 2020, https://www.ft.com/content/a52198f6-0d20-4607-b12a-05110bc48723; J. David Goodman, "How Delays and Unheeded Warnings Hindered New York's Virus Fight," *New York Times*, April 8, 2020, https://www.nytimes.com/2020/04/08/nyregion/new-york-coronavirus-response-delays.html; and Joe Sexton and Joaquin Sapien, "Two Coasts. One Virus. How New York Suffered Nearly 10 Times the Number of Deaths as California," *Pro Publica*, May 16, 2020, https://www.propublica.org/article/two-coasts-one-virus-how-new-york-suffered-nearly-10-times-the-number-of-deaths-as-california.

11. Goodman, "How Delays and Unheeded Warnings Hindered New York's Virus Fight"; and Sexton and Sapien, "Two Coasts."

12. Goodman, "How Delays and Unheeded Warnings Hindered New York's Virus Fight."

13. Damien LaRock, interview by Bridget Bartolini, Queens Memory COVID-19 Project, July 17 and 27, 2020, https://queenslibrary.aviaryplatform.com/collections/943/collection_resources/46728/transcript.

14. Fabio Girelli-Carrasi, "The Angel of Death Over Italy," first published as "From Ground Zero in Italy," Brooklyn College, *Journal of the Plague Year: An Archive of Covid-19*, https://covid-19archive.org/s/archive/item/28432.

15. Re'gan Weal, author interview with Re'gan Weal, March 23, 2023.

16. Ali Mazinov, an early version of this account was written in April 2020 for a class at Brooklyn College taught by Professor Margrethe Horlyck-Romanovsky, archived at Brooklyn College Journal of the Plague Year at https://covid-19archive.org/s/brooklyncollege/item/47989.

17. Keerthan Thiyagarajah interview by Joyce Ma, COVID-19 Asian American Oral History Project, Institutional Archives, LaGuardia Community College, CUNY, December 23, 2021.

18. Davidson Garrett, first published in Mark Nowak, ed., *Coronavirus Haiku: Worker Writers School* (Chicago: Kenning Editions, 2021), 40.

19. Jessica B. Martinez interview conducted by Ryan Hagen for The NYC COVID-19 Oral History, Narrative, and Memory Project, October 13, 2020.

20. Led Black, "The Sirens," first appeared in the Uptown Collective at https://www.uptowncollective.com/2020/04/02/op-led-uptown-love-in-the-time-of-coronavirus-the-sirens/.

21. Steve Zeitlin, "Lamb's Blood." For a discussion of the poem in the larger context of the Passover story, see Caroline Harris and Guest Columnist, "Time All at Once," *Voices: Journal of New York Folklore* 46, no. 1–2 (2020): 22.

2. Working for the Public's Health, Spring 2020

1. Michael Schwirtz, "One Rich N.Y. Hospital Got Warren Buffett's Help, This One Got Duct Tape," *New York Times*, April 26, 2020, https://www.nytimes.com/2020/04/26/nyregion/coronavirus-new-york-university-hospital.html; Brian M. Rosenthal, Joseph Goldstein, Sharon Otterman, and Sheri Fink, "Why Surviving the Virus Might Come Down to Which Hospital Admits You," *New York Times*, July 1, 2020, https://www.nytimes.com/2020/07/01/nyregion/Coronavirus-hospitals.html. On the terrible and dangerous working conditions that essential workers faced in the pandemic, even as they were applauded for their service, see Jamie K. McCallum, *Essential: How the Pandemic Transformed the Long Fight for Worker Justice* (New York: Basic Books, 2022) 5, 8, 10. On the imbalance of hospital bed ratios across the city, see Caleb Melby, Jackie Gu, and Mira Rojanasakul, "Mapping New York City Hospital Beds as Coronavirus Cases Surge," *Bloomberg*, Marcy 25, 2020, updated April 28, 2020, https://www.bloomberg.com/graphics/2020-new-york-coronavirus-outbreak-how-many-hospital-beds/?embedded-checkout=true.

2. Simon Ressner, "Dead on Arrival: A N.Y. Fire Chief's COVID Journal." Early in the pandemic the independent nonprofit news organization Pro Publica asked Simon Ressner of the Fire Department of New York to keep a diary of a twenty-four-hour shift that began at 9:00 a.m. on Friday, April 3, 2020. Published April 5, 2020, at https://www.propublica.org/article/dead-on-arrival-a-ny-fire-chiefs-covid-journal.

3. The New York City Fire Department lost 343 firefighters and paramedics in the attacks of September 11, 2001. See "9/11 By the Numbers," *New York Magazine*, https://nymag.com/news/articles/wtc/1year/numbers.htm.

4. Phil Suarez was interviewed by Rishi Goyal for The NYC COVID-19 Oral History, Narrative, and Memory Project, October 6, 2020.

5. Richard Brea, interviewed by Robert W. Snyder, April 17, 2023.

6. Steven Palmer, interviewed by Mary Marshall Clark for the NYC COVID-19 Oral History, Narrative and Memory Project, June 19, 2020.

7. Patricia Tiu: As a Queens resident and nurse in upper Manhattan, Tiu recorded her observations and posted them on YouTube. Her videos are archived at https://queenslibrary.aviaryplatform.com/collections/943/collection_resources/31398?embed=true.

8. Christopher Tedeschi, interviewed by Denise Milstein for the NYC COVID-19 Oral History, Narrative and Memory Project, July 14th, 2020.

9. "Richard Jenkins" is a pseudonym. Interviewed by Ryan Hagen for the NYC COVID-19 Oral History, Narrative, and Memory Project, May 7, 2020.

10. Steven Palmer, interviewed by Robert W. Snyder, March 4, 2023.

3. Work Turned Upside Down, Spring to Fall 2020

1. Christina Goldbaum, "41 Transit Workers Dead; Crisis Takes Staggering Toll on Subways," *New York Times*, April 8, 2020, https://www.nytimes.com/2020/04/08/nyregion/coronavirus-nyc-mta-subway.html.

2. Goldbaum, "41 Transit Workers Dead."

3. Re'gan Weal, interviewed by Robert W. Snyder, March 23, 2023.

4. Ralph Rolle, interviewed by Bethany Fernandez for the Bronx COVID-19 Oral History Project of Fordham University, July 26, 2020, https://www.thebronxcovid19oralhistoryproject.com/interviews/ralph-rolle.

5. Elizabeth Petrillo, interviewed by Anthony Brognano for the Staten Island Coronavirus Chronicle Oral History Project at the College of Staten Island, May 19, 2021.

6. Patricia Hernandez, interviewed by Veronica Quiroga for the Bronx COVID-19 Oral History Project of Fordham University, May 10, 2020, https://www.thebronxcovid19oralhistoryproject.com/interviews/patricia-hernandez.

7. Maribel Gonzalez Christianson, interviewed by Bethany Fernandez for the Bronx COVID-19 Oral History Project of Fordham University, June 2, 2020, https://www.thebronxcovid19oralhistoryproject.com/interviews/maribel-gonzalez.

8. Gustavo Ajche, interviewed by Martha Guerrero Badillo, November 1, 2021.

9. Claudia Irizarry Aponte, Josefa Velasquez, and Katie Honan, "New York City Passes Landmark New Protections for Food Delivery Workers," *THE CITY*, September 23, 2–21, https://www.thecity.nyc/2021/09/23/new-york-city-landmark-food-delivery-worker-law/.

10. Damien LaRock, interviewed by Bridget Bartolini, Queens Memory COVID-19 Project, July 17 and 27, 2020, https://queenslibrary.aviaryplatform.com/collections/943/collection_resources/46728/transcript.

11. Rachel Hadas' poem "In the Cloud" first appeared in *The New Yorker* and was also published in Hadas's book *Pandemic Almanac* (Princeton, NJ: Ragged Sky Press, 2022).

12. Beth Evans, excerpted from Beth Evans, "Inside and Outside, At Home," *Journal of the Plague Year: An Archive of Covid-19*, Brooklyn College (spring 2020), https://covid-19archive.org/s/archive/item/30688.

13. Robert Kelley, interviewed by Robert W. Snyder, January 24, 2023.

4. Losses, Spring 2020

1. On the pattern of deaths, see "Trends and Totals," https://www.nyc.gov/site/doh/covid/covid-19-data-totals.page.

2. See "Funeral and Burial Guidance," https://www.nyc.gov/site/help-nownyc/get-help/funeral-burial-guidance.page.

3. Author communication with Rachel Hadas, August 31, 2023.

4. "Health Advisory: COVID-19 Guidance for Hospital Operators Regarding Visitation," New York State Department of Health, March 18, 2020, https://coronavirus.health.ny.gov/system/files/documents/2020/03/doh_covid19_obpedsvisitation_032720.pdf.

5. For photographs of hospital staff and a chaplain tending to patients in extreme conditions, see "Collection on COVID-19" at the Mount Sinai Health System (AA119). The Arthur H. Aufses, Jr. MD Archives, Icahn School of Medicine at Mount Sinai/Mount Sinai Health System, New York, NY. On the extremely difficult conditions that confronted health care professionals, see Marie Brenner, *The Desperate Hours: One Hospital's Fight to Save a City on the Pandemic's Front Lines* (New York: Flatiron Books, 2022), 249–55, 260, 275–76; Schwirtz, "One Rich N.Y. Hospital"; Rosenthal, Goldstein, Otterman, and Fink, "Why Surviving."

6. W. J. Hennigan, "'We Do This for the Living': Inside New York's Citywide Effort to Bury Its Dead," *Time*, May 21, 2020, https://time.com/5839056/new-york-city-burials-coronavirus/.

7. "Funeral and Burial Guidance," HELP NOW NYC.

8. Stephanie McCrummen, "Death Without Ritual," *Washington Post*, April 4, 2020, https://www.washingtonpost.com/nation/2020/04/04/funeral-home-new-york-city-bodies-coronavirus/.

9. The poem by Alfred Small first appeared in Mark Nowak, ed., *Coronavirus Haiku: Worker Writers School* (Chicago: Kenning Editions, 2021), 33.

10. The poem by Thomas Barzey first appeared in Nowak, ed., *Coronavirus Haiku*, 85.

11. Nichole Matos, interviewed by Veronica Quiroga for the Bronx COVID-19 Oral History Project of Fordham University, April 26, 2020, https://www.library.fordham.edu/digital/item/collection/bxcvdoralhist/id/4.

12. Copy of letter in author's possession.

13. Rozelyn Murray first published this essay in *COVID Class 2021*, a platform for students in David Rohlfing's English 12 class at Pace High School.

14. Michèle Voltaire Marcelin: Published here with permission of the author.

15. C.A. Duran, this essay first appeared in *COVID Class 2021*, a platform for students in David Rohlfing's English 12 class at Pace High School.

16. Robert W. Snyder interview with Veronica E. Fletcher, February 5, 2023.

5. Coping, Spring 2020

1. Jeremy Berke, "'We Are Flattening the Curve': Cuomo Says Shutdowns Are Working to Curb the Spread of the Coronavirus, but It's 'Not a Time to Get Complacent,'" *Business Insider*, April 8, 2020, https://www.business insider.com/coronavirus-cuomo-says-new-york-flattening-the-curve-2020–4; Jeffrey E. Harris, "The Coronavirus Epidemic Curve Is Already Flattening in New York City," National Bureau of Economic Research, April 2020, https://www.nber. org/papers/w26917.

2. Jesse McKinley and Shane Goldmacher, "How Cuomo, Once on Sidelines, Became the Politician of the Moment," *New York Times*, March 24, 2020, https:// www.nytimes.com/2020/03/24/nyregion/governor-andrew-cuomo-coronavi- rus.html; Bill Hammond, *2020 Hindsight: Rebuilding New York's Public Health Defenses After the Coronavirus Pandemic* (Albany: Empire Center, 2021), 8–13, 19–24.

3. On Cuomo, de Blasio, and their uneven responses to the pandemic, see J. David Goodman, "How Delays and Unheeded Warnings Hindered New York's Virus Fight," *New York Times*, April 8, 2020, https://www.nytimes. com/2020/04/08/nyregion/new-york-coronavirus-response-delays.html; Shalini Ramachandran, Laura Kusisto, and Katie Homan, "How New York's Corona- virus Response Made the Pandemic Worse," *Wall Street Journal*, June 11, 2020, https://www.wsj.com/articles/how-new-yorks-coronavirus-response-made-the- pandemic-worse-11591908426; Hannah Kuchler, "How New York's Missteps Let Covid-19 Overwhelm the US," *Financial Times*, October 2, 2020, https://www. ft.com/content/a52198f6-0d20-4607-b12a-05110bc48723; Joe Sexton and Joa- quin Sapien, "Two Coasts, One Virus," *Pro Publica*, May 16, 2020, https://www. propublica.org/article/two-coasts-one-virus-how-new-york-suffered-nearly- 10-times-the-number-of-deaths-as-california; and Hammond, *2020 Hindsight*, 8–13, 19–24.

4. Liam Stack, "De Blasio Breaks Up Rabbi's Funeral and Lashes Out Over Virus Distancing," *New York Times*, April 28, 2020, https://www.nytimes. com/2020/04/28/nyregion/hasidic-funeral-coronavirus-de-blasio.html; Sander L. Gilman, "Placing the Blame for Covid-19 in and on Ultra-Orthodox Com- munities," *Modern Judaism*, December 30, 2020, https://doi.org/10.1093/mj/ kjaa021; Josefa Velazquez, Ann Choi, and Clifford Michel, "Southern Brooklyn's Ongoing COVID Suffering Shows Toll of Disinformation and Disconnection," *The City*, May 26, 2021, https://www.thecity.nyc/2021/05/26/southern-brooklyn- covid-death-disinformation-disconnection/. On uneven adherence to masking

and police responses to masking requirements, see Michael Wilson, "At Least New Yorkers Can Still Roll Their Eyes," *New York Times*, April 17, 2020, https://www.nytimes.com/2020/04/17/nyregion/new-york-coronavirus-masks.html; Tina Moore, Julia Marsh, Bernadette Hogan, Nolan Hicks, and Aaron Feis, "NYPD Blows Off Concerns over Cops Ditching Masks during Coronavirus," *New York Post*, June 11, 2020, https://nypost.com/2020/06/11/nypd-blows-off-concerns-over-cops-ditching-coronavirus-masks/; Michael Wilson, "Why Are So Many N.Y.P.D. Officers Refusing to Wear Masks at Protests?" *New York Times*, June 11, 2020, https://www.nytimes.com/2020/06/11/nyregion/nypd-face-masks-nyc-protests.html; and Andy Newman, "Are New Yorkers Wearing Masks? Here's What We Found in Each Borough," *New York Times*, August 20, 2020, https://www.nytimes.com/2020/08/20/nyregion/nyc-face-masks.html.

5. Alexandra E. Petri and Daniel E. Slotnik, "Attacks on Asian-Americans in New York Stoke Fear, Anxiety, and Anger," *New York Times*, February 26, 2021, https://www.nytimes.com/2021/02/26/nyregion/asian-hate-crimes-attacks-ny.html; Weyi Cai, Audra D.S. Burch, and Jugal K. Patel, "Swelling Anti-Asian Violence: Who Is Being Attacked Where," *New York Times*, April 3, 2021, https://www.nytimes.com/interactive/2021/04/03/us/anti-asian-attacks.html; ADL, *Hate in the Empire State: Extremism and Antisemitism in New York*, 2020–2021, May 19, 2022, https://www.adl.org/resources/report/hate-empire-state-extremism-anti-semitism-new-york-2020-2021.

6. Mackenzie Kwok: With permission of the author.

7. Trends and totals: https://www.nyc.gov/site/doh/covid/covid-19-data-totals.page.

8. Davidson Garrett: Mark Nowak, ed., *Coronavirus Haiku: Worker Writers School* (Chicago: Kenning Editions, 2021), 40.

9. Adele Dressner: An earlier version of this essay appeared in *Sounds I Never Heard Before: Reflections on the COVID-19 Pandemic*, a zine published in August 2020 by the Lasting Impressions Department of DOROT, a Manhattan organization founded to improve the lives and health of older adults.

10. Sumya Abida: With permission of the author. Thanks to Steve Zeitlin for introducing Sumya Abida and her work to the editor.

11. An earlier version of Matilda Virgilio Clark's essay appeared in *Sounds I Never Heard Before: Reflections on the COVID-19 Pandemic*, a zine published in August 2020 by the Lasting Impressions Department of DOROT, a Manhattan organization founded to improve the lives and health of older adults.

12. Reprinted with the permission of Ron Kolm, a contributing editor of *Sensitive Skin Magazine*, the author of five books of poetry and two collections of short fictions, and the editor of six *Unbearables* anthologies.

13. Reprinted with the permission of the author.

14. Kleber Vera (Flame), interviewed by Oscar Zamora Flores for the Queens Memory Project, January 13, 2021, https://queenslibrary.aviaryplatform.com/col-

lections/943/collection_resources/39882/transcript?u=t&keywords[]=Kleber& keywords[]=Vera.

15. Sheikh Musa Drammeh, interviewed by Dr. Jane Kani Edward and Bethany Fernandez for the Bronx COVID-19 Oral History Project at Fordham University, October 7, 2020, https://www.thebronxcovid19oralhistoryproject.com/interviews/sheikh-musa-drammeh.

16. Keerthan Thiyagarajah, interviewed by Joyce Ma, COVID-19 Asian American Oral History Project, Institutional Archives, LaGuardia Community College, CUNY, December 23, 2021.

17. Dave Crenshaw, interviewed by Robert W. Snyder, May 11, 2023.

18. Reprinted from the *Uptown Collective*, https://www.uptowncollective.com/2020/04/17/op-led-uptown-love-in-the-time-of-coronavirus-clap-because-you-care/.

6. Opening Up, Summer and Fall 2020

1. Margaret Garnett, commissioner, *Investigations into NYPD Response to the George Floyd Protests* (New York City: NY City Department of Investigation, December 2020); New York City Civilian Complaint Review Board, *2020 NYC Protests* (February 6, 2023), https://www.nyc.gov/site/ccrb/policy/issue-based-reports.page; and *NYPD Response to CCRB's "2020 Protest Report,"* https://www.nyc.gov/site/nypd/news/p00074/nypd-response-ccrb-s-2020-protest-report-.

2. Susan Sachs, "Giuliani's Goal of Civil City Runs Into First Amendment," *New York Times*, July 6, 1998, https://www.nytimes.com/1998/07/06/nyregion/giuliani-s-goal-of-civil-city- runs-into-first-amendment.html; Ben Adler, "Bloomberg's Long War Against Protests," *CityLab*, November 16, 2011, https://www.bloomberg.com/news/articles/2011-11-16/bloomberg-s-long-war-against-protests; Conor Friedersdorf, "What Bloomberg Did to Peaceful Protesters," *The Atlantic*, February 25, 2020, https://www.theatlantic.com/ideas/archive/2020/02/what-bloomberg-did-rnc-protesters/607030/.

3. Christina Goldbaum, Liam Stack, and Alex Traub, "After Peaceful Protests, Looters Strike at Macy's and Across Midtown," *New York Times*, June 2, 2020, https://www.nytimes.com/2020/06/02/nyregion/nyc-looting-protests.html; Azi Paybarah and Nikita Stewart, "Symbol of N.Y.C. Unrest: A Burning Police Car," *New York Times*, May 31, 2020, https://www.nytimes.com/2020/05/31/nyregion/police-cars-nyc-protests.html; Ali Watkins, "An Unprepared N.Y.P.D. Badly Mishandled Floyd Protests, Watchdog Says," *New York Times*, Dec. 18, 2020, https://www.nytimes.com/2020/12/18/nyregion/nypd-george-floyd-protests.html; John Bolger, "Exclusive: NYPD Took Hours to Respond to Mass Looting, Despite Quickly Cracking Down on Protests," *The Intercept*, June 1, 2021, https://theintercept.com/2021/06/01/nypd-looting-violence-protest/. Maura Grunlund, "'Let Staten Island Be an Example'—As City Burned, Peaceful Protests over

George Floyd Here," June 1, 2020, https://www.silive.com/news/2020/06/let-staten-island-be-an-example-as-city-burned-peaceful-protests-over-george-floyd-here.html.

4. See Peter Senzamici, "Anger and Demand for Answers as Cops Seem to 'Deputize' Inwood Anti-Looting Posse," *The City*, June 12, 2020, https://www.thecity.nyc/2020/06/12/demand-for-answers-as-inwood-cops-seem-to-deputize-anti-looting-posse/. For police speaking with local men about safeguarding the neighborhood, see https://www.youtube.com/watch?v=6AswojkjYw&t=331s; for local men patrolling the streets, see https://www.youtube.com/watch?v=7Ee24Vf-K2A.

5. Mariame Kaba, "Yes, We Mean Literally Abolish the Police," *New York Times*, June 12, 2020, https://www.nytimes.com/2020/06/12/opinion/sunday/floyd-abolish-defund-police.html.

6. Colin Moynihan, "New York to Pay $13 Million Over Police Actions at George Floyd Protests," *New York Times*, July 20, 2023, https://www.nytimes.com/2023/07/20/nyregion/nypd-george-floyd-protesters-settlement.html.

7. Gregory Neyman and Willliam Dalsey, "Black Lives Matter Protests and COVID-19 Cases: Relationship in Two Databases," *Journal of Public Health* (November 2020), https://www.ncbi.nlm.nih.gov/pmc/articles/PMC77 17330/.

8. Andy Newman, "Are New Yorkers Wearing Masks? Here's What We Found in Each Borough," *New York Times*, August 8, 2020, https://www.nytimes.com/2020/08/20/nyregion/nyc-face-masks.html.

9. Christina Goldbaum, "When a Bus Driver Told a Rider to Wear a Mask, 'He Knocked Me Out Cold,'" *New York Times*, September 18, 2020, https://www.nytimes.com/2020/09/18/nyregion/mta-bus-mask-covid.html?action=click&module=Top%20Stories&pgtype=Homepage.

10. Amanda Rosa, "How a Bar Became a Symbol of Staten Island Virus Defiance," *New York Times*, December 9, 2020, https://www.nytimes.com/2020/12/09/nyregion/macs-staten-island-covid.html#:~:text=The%20bar%20flouted%20a%20curfew,rates%2C%20the%20bar%20stayed%20open; and Eric Klinenberg, *2020: One City, Seven People, and the Year Everything Changed* (New York: Alfred A. Knopf, 2024) 118-137.

11. Luis Ferré-Sadurní and Joseph Goldstein, "1st Vaccination in U.S. Is Given in New York, Hard Hit in Outbreak's First Days," *New York Times*, December 14, 2020, https://www.nytimes.com/2020/12/14/nyregion/coronavirus-vaccine-new-york.html.

12. Thomas Barzey in Mark Nowak, ed., *Coronavirus Haiku: Worker Writers School* (Chicago: Kenning Editions, 2021), 66.

13. Published with permission of the author.

14. Richard Brea, interviewed by Robert W. Snyder, April 17, 2023.

15. Alexandra L. Naranjo, interviewed by Stephanie Khalifa for the Staten Island Coronavirus Chronicle Oral History Project at the College of Staten Island, May 16, 2021.

16. Kleber Vera (Flame), interviewed by Oscar Zamora Flores for the Queens Memory Project, January 13, 2021, https://queenslibrary.aviaryplatform.com/collections/943/collection_resources/39882/transcript?u=t&keywords[]=Kleber&keywords[]=Vera.

17. Patricia Tiu, interviewed by Jamie Beckenstein of the Queens Memory Project, June 11, 2020, https://queenslibrary.aviaryplatform.com/collections/943/collection_resources/31398/file/123688/transcript?embed=true.

18. Keerthan Thiyagarajah, interviewed by Joyce Ma, December 23, 2021, for the COVID-19 Asian American Oral History Project, Institutional Archives, LaGuardia Community College, CUNY.

19. Phil Suarez, interviewed by Rishi Goyal for the NYC COVID-19 Oral History, Narrative and Memory Project, October 6, 2020.

20. Richard Jenkins (a pseudonym), interviewed by Ryan Hagen for the NYC COVID-19 Oral History, Narrative, and Memory Project, May 7, 2020.

21. Jessica B. Martinez, interviewed by Ryan Hagen for the NYC COVID-19 Oral History, Narrative, and Memory Project, October 13, 2020.

22. Maribel Gonzalez Christianson, interviewed by Bethany Fernandez for the Bronx COVID-19 Oral History Project, November 11, 2020.

23. Jessica B. Martinez, interviewed by Ryan Hagen for the NYC COVID-19 Oral History, Narrative and Memory Project, March 3, 2021. For a description of festivities, see Edgar Sandoval, "A Rollicking N.Y. C. Celebration for Biden's Win, Well Into the Night," *New York Times*, November 7, 2020, https://www.nytimes.com/2020/11/07/nyregion/nyc-reaction-biden-win.html.

7. Vaccines and After, 2021

1. Quoted in Edith Wharton, *French Ways and Their Meaning* (London: Macmillan, 1909), 65.

2. Luis Ferré-Sadurní and Joseph Goldstein "1st Vaccination in U.S. Is Given in New York, Hard Hit in Outbreak's First Days," *New York Times*, December 14, 2020, https://www.nytimes.com/2020/12/14/nyregion/coronavirus-vaccine-new-york.html.

3. Shira Ovide, "The Problem With Vaccine Websites," *New York Times*, January 12, 2021, https://www.nytimes.com/2021/01/12/technology/the-problem-with-vaccine-websites.html; S. Mitra Kalita, "What We Learned Registering Thousands of Our Neighbors for Vaccines," *Epicenter-NYC*, March 22, 2021, https://epicenter-nyc.com/what-we-learned-registering-thousands-of-our-neighbors-for-vaccines/.

4. Deepti Hajela and Michael R. Sisak, "NYC Honors Essential Workers at Parade up Canyon of Heroes," *Associated Press*, July 7, 2021, https://

apnews.com/article/lifestyle-parades-canyons-coronavirus-pandemic-health-f6fbcd3b911164a6bcc9c51ca1fb5563; Mihir Zaveri and Ashley Wong, "Why Some of N.Y.C.'s Essential Workers Skipped a Parade to Honor Them," *New York Times*, July 7, 2021, https://www.nytimes.com/2021/07/07/nyregion/NYC-parade-essential-workers.html.

5. Paul A. Offitt, M.D., Foreword in *Deadly Choices: How the Anti-Vaccine Movement Threatens Us All* (New York: Basic Books, 2015); Elena Conis, *Vaccine Nation: America's Changing Relationship with Immunization* (Chicago: University of Chicago Press, 2014).

6. Jake Offenharz, "'This Is Tyranny': NYC Municipal Workers March On City Hall To Protest COVID Vaccine Mandate," *Gothamist*, October 25, 2021, https://gothamist.com/news/tyranny-nyc-municipal-workers-march-city-hall-protest-covid-vaccine-mandate.

7. Anita Sreedhar and Anand Gopal, "Behind Low Vaccination Rates Lurks a More Profound Social Weakness," *New York Times*, December 3, 2021, https://www.nytimes.com/2021/12/03/opinion/vaccine-hesitancy-covid.html. Also see Caitjan Ganty, "The US Once withheld Syphilis Treatment from Hundreds of Black Men in the Name of Science," *The Conversation*, January 12, 2024, https://theconversation.com/the-us-once-withheld-syphilis-treatment-from-hundreds-of-black-men-in-the-name-of-science-newly-public-records-are-helping-us-understand-how-it-could-happen-217216; Vanessa Northington Gamble, "Under the Shadow of Tuskegee: African Americans and Health Care," *American Journal of Public Health* 87, no. 11 (November 1997), https://pubmed.ncbi.nlm.nih.gov/9366634/; and Carrie D. Wollinetz, PhD, and Francis S. Collins, MD, PhD, "Recognition of Research Participants' Need for Autonomy: Remembering the Legacy of Henrietta Lacks," *Journal of the American Medical Association*, August 11, 2020, 1027–28, https://jamanetwork.com/journals/jama/fullarticle/2769506. On vaccination rates, see Nambi Ndugga, Latoya Hill, Samantha Artiga, and Sweta Haldar, "Latest Data on COVID-19 Vaccination by Race/Ethnicity," *KFF*, July 14, 2022, https://www.kff.org/coronavirus-covid-19/issue-brief/latest-data-on-covid-19-vaccinations-by-race-ethnicity/.

8. Emma G. Fitzsimmons, Joseph Goldstein and Sharon Otterman, "New York City Mandates Vaccines for Its Workers to 'End the Covid Era,'" *New York Times*, October 20, 2021, https://www.nytimes.com/2021/10/20/nyregion/nyc-vaccine-mandate.html; Joseph Goldstein and Sharon Otterman, "9,000 Unvaccinated N.Y.C. Workers Put on Unpaid Leave as Mandate Begins," *New York Times*, November 1, 2021, https://www.nytimes.com/2021/11/01/nyregion/nyc-vaccine-mandate.html. On transit workers, see Clayton Guse, "MTA becomes one of NYC's least vaccinated public workforces," *Daily News*, November 2, 2021, https://www.nydailynews.com/2021/11/02/mta-becomes-one-of-nycs-least-vaccinated-public-workforces/.

9. ADL, *Hate in the Empire State: Extremism and Antisemitism in New York, 2020–2021*, May 19, 2022, https://www.adl.org/resources/report/hate-empire-state-extremism-antisemitism-new-york-2020–2021.

10. See citywide total of shooting victims in New York City Police Department, *CompStat YEAR END 2020 FINAL* (January 14, 2021), 30.

11. Shannon Young, "Timeline: Countdown to Cuomo's Downfall," *Politico*, August 3, 2021, https://www.politico.com/states/new-york/albany/story/2021/08/03/timeline-countdown-to-cuomos-downfall-1389414; Yoav Gonen, "Eric Adams Wins NYC Mayoral Election, Earning His Chance to Make History in Post-COVID Era, "*The City*, November 2, 2021, https://www.thecity.nyc/2021/11/02/eric-adams-wins-nyc-mayoral-election-leading-in-covid-era/.

12. Justin Fox, "New York, I Love You, But You're Bringing Me Down," *Bloomberg Opinion*, March 9, 2023, https://www.bloomberg.com/graphics/2023-opinion-how-livable-are-cities-three-years-after-start-of-covid/new-york-city.html.

13. Dave Crenshaw, interviewed by Robert W. Snyder, May 11, 2023.

14. Rachel Hadas, "The Second Shot," *Pandemic Almanac* (Princeton, NJ: Ragged Sky Press, 2022), 58.

15. Alexandra L. Naranjo, interviewed by Stephanie Khalifa for the Staten Island Coronavirus Chronicle Oral History Project at the College of Staten Island, May 16, 2021.

16. Christopher Tedeschi, interviewed by Denise Milstein for The NYC COVID-19 Oral History, Narrative and Memory Project, January 25, 2021.

17. Jessica B. Martinez, interviewed by Ryan Hagen for The NYC COVID-19 Oral History, Narrative and Memory Archive, March 3, 2021.

18. "Lexicon of the Pandemic" appeared first in *Covid Class 2021*, a platform for students in David Rohlfing's English 12 class at Pace High School.

19. Mackenzie Kwok, "The Bitterness I Eat," was written and performed for Annie Lanzillotto's virtual talk show, *Tell Me a Story*.

20. Steve Zeitlin, "The Island of Pandemica," Published with permission of the author.

8. Reflections, 2023

1. Lena H. Sun and Amy Goldstein, "What the End of the COVID Public Health Emergency Means for You," *Washington Post*, May 4, 2023, https://www.washingtonpost.com/health/2023/05/04/covid-public-health-emergency-end/; and Kathy Katella, "3 Things to Know About JN.1, the New Coronavirus Strain," *Yale Medicine*, January 31, 2024, https://www.yalemedicine.org/news/jn1-coronavirus-variant-covid.

2. N. P. Johnson and J. Mueller, "Updating the Accounts: Global Mortality of the 1918–1920 'Spanish' Influenza Pandemic," *Bulletin of the History of Medicine* 76, no. 1 (2002): 105–15, doi:10.1353/bhm.2002.0022. Figures on the death toll of the flu in New York City vary. Francesco Aimone's figure of thirty thousand includes deaths from both flu and pneumonia, a common combination of illnesses that contributed to the deadly nature of the flu. See Francesco Aimone,

"The 1918 Influenza Epidemic in New York City: A Review of the Public Health Response," *Public Health Reports* volume 125, Supplement 3 (2010): 71–79. Useful books on the flu epidemic of 1918 include Alfred W. Crosby, *America's Forgotten Pandemic: The Influenza of 1918* (New York: Cambridge University Press, 2003); and Laura Spinney, *Pale Rider: The Spanish Flu and How it Changed the World* (New York: Public Affairs, 2017).

3. Dave Crenshaw, interviewed by Robert W. Snyder, April 17, 2023.

4. Richard Brea, interviewed by Robert W. Snyder, April 17, 2023.

5. Re'gan Weal, interviewed by Robert W. Snyder, March 23, 2023.

6. Veronica E. Fletcher, interviewed by Robert W. Snyder, March 23, 2023.

7. Steven Palmer, interviewed by Robert W. Snyder, March 4, 2023.

8. Keerthan Thiyagarajah, interviewed by Joyce Ma for the COVID-19 Asian American Oral History Project at LaGuardia Community College, CUNY, December 23, 2021.

Conclusion

1. Paul Starr, "Reckoning with National Failure: The Case of Covid," *Liberties* 1, no 3 (spring 2021): 73.

2. Klinenberg, *2020,* 366–69. The point on the interdependence of strangers was once made by the late Michael Harrington, citing Karl Marx.

Contributors

Interviewees

Gustavo Ajche, bicycle courier

Richard Brea, New York City Police Department, retired

Maribel Gonzalez Christianson, owner, The South of France restaurant

Dave Crenshaw, community coach

Sheikh Musa Drammeh, founder of the Islamic Leadership School and the Muslim Media Corporation and CEO of Halalfinder.com

Veronica E. Fletcher, former teacher

Patricia Hernandez, sales clerk and student at John Jay College

Richard Jenkins, medical doctor, New York City (pseudonym)

Robert Kelley, vice president, Local 100, Transport Workers Union

Damien LaRock, special education teacher, PS 148, Queens

Jessica B. Martinez, global health expert

Nichole Matos, John Jay College of Criminal Justice student and gym worker

Alexandra L. Naranjo, client advocate

Steven Palmer, physician assistant and clinical coordinator, HIV vaccines unit, Columbia University Medical Center

Elizabeth Petrillo, cashier and student, St. John's University

Ralph Rolle, musician, producer, and co-owner and proprietor of the Soul Snacks Cookie Company

Phil Suarez, paramedic, humanitarian aid worker, and a photographer

Christopher Tedeschi, emergency physician, Columbia Medical Center and Allen Hospital

Keerthan Thiyagarajah, LaGuardia Community College student and cook

Patricia Tiu, nurse, NewYork–Presbyterian/Weill Cornell Medical Center

Kleber Vera (Flame), hairstylist and LGBT activist

Re'gan Weal, bus operator, MTA New York City Transit

Interviewers

Bridget Bartolini, Queens Memory Project, Queens Public Library

Jamie Beckenstein, Queens Memory Project, Queens Public Library

Anthony Brognano, Lockdown Staten Island, College of Staten Island

Mary Marshall Clark, NYC COVID-19 Oral History, Narrative, and Memory Project; and director, Columbia Center for Oral History Research

Dr. Jane Kani Edward, Bronx COVID-19 Oral History Project, Fordham University

Bethany Fernandez, Bronx COVID-19 Oral History Project, Fordham University

Rishi Goyal, NYC COVID-19 Oral History, Narrative, and Memory Project

Martha Guerrero Badillo, doctoral student, History Department, Yale University

Ryan Hagen, NYC COVID-19 Oral History, Narrative, and Memory Project

Stephanie Khalifa, Lockdown Staten Island, College of Staten Island

Joyce Ma, COVID-19 Asian American Oral History Project, LaGuardia Community College

Denise Milstein, NYC COVID-19 Oral History, Narrative, and Memory Project

Veronica Quiroga, Bronx COVID-19 Oral History Project, Fordham University

Oscar Zamora Flores, Queens Memory Project, Queens Public Library

Poets

Thomas Barzey, actor

Davidson Garrett, poet, writer, and actor

Rachel Hadas, professor emeritus of English at Rutgers University–Newark, poet, author, and translator

Ron Kolm, poet, editor, and author

Michèle Voltaire Marcelin, poet, visual artist, and performer

Alfreda Small, retired home health aide and police administrator

Steve Zeitlin, folklorist, writer, cultural activist, author of twelve books on America's folk culture

Writers

Sumya Abida, student, Bard High School Early College, Manhattan

Led Black, founder and editor-in-chief of www.uptowncollective.com

Lily M. Chin, knit and crochet designer and instructor

Matilda Virgilio Clark, seamstress, babysitter, house cleaner, administrative assistant, and life coach

Adele Dressner, president, All-In-One Suppliers, retired
C. A. Duran, student, Pace High School
Beth Evans, associate professor and librarian, Brooklyn College
Fabio Girelli-Carasi, professor, Brooklyn College
David Hunt, **Tess McDade**, and **Peter Walsh**, proprietors, Coogan's Bar and Restaurant
Mackenzie Kwok, folklorist and singer-songwriter
Ali Mazinov, Brooklyn College student and paramedic
Rozelyn Murray, student, Pace High School
Clifford Pearson, writer and urbanist
Simon Ressner, New York City firefighter

Photographers

Kevin J. Call, MTA New York City Transit
Patrick Cashin, MTA New York City Transit
Megan Green
Marc A. Hermann, MTA New York City Transit
Nicholas Knight
Erica Lansner
Paul Margolis
Erik McGregor
James Melchiorre
John Minchillo, Associated Press
Tom Pich
Naima Rauam
Arlene Schulman
Alon Sicherman and **Sean Vegezzi**, The Hart Island Project
Bryan R. Smith
Josue Tepancal Jimenez

Index